The Paradigm of Happiness

By

Jack Lafayette

Table of Contents

Introduction

Waking up is especially difficult today. The alarm rings once. I hit the snooze button *hard*. The last thing I want to hear is the chirpy, upbeat ringtone of my alarm. Rolling over, I doze off again for another five minutes before the snooze alarm rings again.

Ugh! I feel around for my smartphone and wish I could sleep in just a little longer. It's that kind of day already. The kind that I just don't want to face.

Maybe you've been there, too. Just getting out of bed can be hard. It gets worse when you pull the curtain and outside the weather looks gloomy and gray. Going to the bathroom and looking at yourself in the mirror doesn't make things any better, either.

Traffic is slow on the way to work. People just don't seem to know how to drive well these days. As you pass by another fender bender, now fifteen minutes late to work, you wish you could just turn around and climb back into bed.

Still, things have changed. With the Covid-19 pandemic looming, many people have had to learn how to work from home. At first, the idea of being able to catch a few more Zs seems great. Being able to take your time making breakfast and having a cup of coffee brewing seems heavenly. Day after day, though, the reality of working at home begins to take its toll.

For some, working at home means struggling to juggle your kids and their school with your work. It means bringing the stress of work into your home. It means feeling more trapped than ever without having the option or space to relax. It means learning new ways of interacting with loved ones online and navigating even more input from social media than before.

Whether you can go to work or have to remain at home, I am sure you are facing new challenges every day. Sometimes, you can overcome. Sometimes, you might have felt like a loser. I know that I have gone on a real rollercoaster ride thanks to Covid-19. Over time, I realized that I was slowly being drained of energy and inspiration. Negative feelings and ideas began to pile up.

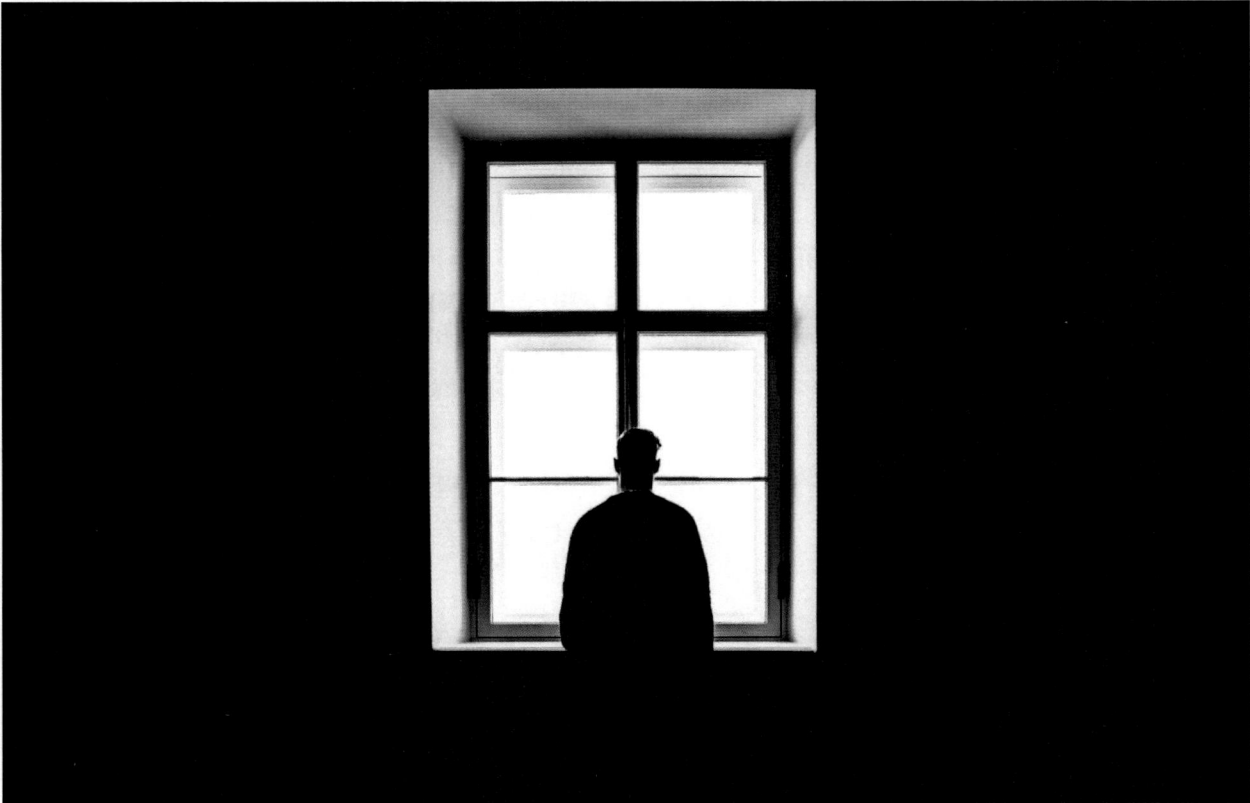

Isolated. Although the internet is useful in the many ways it connects people, time on Zoom is never the same as time spent face-to-face with someone. Even when I was able to meet up with my friend, I was still confronted by this strange new reality we were both living in. I never felt so happy hanging with my friend and so disconnected at the same time

Overwhelmed. If feeling alone wasn't bad enough, whenever I hopped online to check Instagram posts or Snapchat stories, I felt bombarded by everything I saw. So many opinions, rumors, and opposing views. It was a never-ending flood of information. People always seem to be fighting online, unable to listen to each other and learn. Social media these days feels both frustrating and comforting.

Stressed. The news and stories my friends tell me aren't much better than what I see on the internet. With all the statistics for the virus coming in, political tension around the world rising, and concerns about job stability, it's hard not to get stressed out. I know that my friends and family are struggling as well, but I don't know how to help them much less help myself. What am I supposed to do?

Restricted. Even though I have a few ideas about what I need to destress and reconnect with myself and my life, I feel like my options right now are limited. With contradictory information coming through news and social media, I'm not sure what I can and cannot do. How can I reconnect with nature? How can I take care of myself? How can I maintain interest in daily life?

Unmotivated. The lack of motivation is real. Even if I find some time for peace and quiet, when I sit down in front of my laptop I find it hard to focus on work. Even trying to find new hobbies or skills leaves me in a numb, lack of motivation state.

Empty. Without the creative juices flowing, my home-care and self-care suffer. Unable to express myself, I feel like a negative loop of emotional emptiness has been created. I feel empty. I'm not able to work through my difficulties by achieving small goals, and since I am unable to accomplish anything, I feel even more inadequate than ever. With social isolation making me feel this way, I just want to put my feet up and veg out.

Finding Answers

Once I listed all of these negative emotions that I would experience on any day, I knew that something had to change. I knew that there had to be options out there for me to explore. This wasn't the time to give up. Instead of seeing it as a rescue, I reframed this as my fight for self-care and self-compassion. This was a chance for me to rise to the challenge and become stronger in the face of these difficulties. The truth was that I had to accept the things I couldn't change and figure out what things I could change. I knew I could mature and rise to meet the challenges.

As I experimented, I discovered what worked for me and what didn't. I realized that happiness is achieved through small life changes. *Great transformations take time.* The small steps I set as goals for myself not only moved me closer to my long-term goals of happiness and mental health but also increased my self-confidence and self-determination. In this book, I'm going to share what worked for me—the small practical steps that you can start on today!

Chapter 1:

My Quiet Time

Are you the parent who always feels run-down and overworked at home? Your house feels too cluttered. Everything seems to be a perpetual mess. The idea of achieving a deep clean seems impossible at this point. You barely have time to crack open a window! Part of the reason why things are so out of control is that your kids haven't been able to get a solid year of school. In between confusing Zoom call sessions with their classes, they struggle to focus on their classwork and end up making more of a mess around the house. It just feels like a disaster you cannot escape.

Or are you the single who is struggling with motivation and loneliness? At first, the idea of spending time alone is appealing. The more relaxed pace of working from home is a nice change of pace. However, as time goes on, the isolation gets to you, or you begin to lose the more active, healthier habits you maintained. Before you know it, you are staying up late, munching on snacks, and chilling with Netflix or gaming with friends online. You find yourself sleeping in. Focusing on work becomes more difficult, and you never reach your deadlines on time. Lack of motivation and concentration combined with phone distractions are eating away at your creativity. You begin to wonder if there is any way to get yourself going every day.

What if you have the opposite problem? Bringing work home has just amped up the pressure to perform. Whether you have a boss that does not respect boundaries or you struggle with workaholic tendencies, you might find yourself at a loss in drawing a line between personal space and workspace. Swallowed by your job, you might find it hard to set time aside for yourself. Even if you manage to start the day off on a good foot, you might work through lunch and forget to eat. Stuck in the zone, thinking"I just need to get one more thing done", you find yourself working 10 hours a day. If your at-home office is stuck in the corner of your bedroom, the ability to walk away from work might become more difficult than ever. Is there a way to recover your own life?

All of these scenarios are complex. You may end up having to use a variety of solutions in order to cope with these kinds of difficulties. The good news is that many answers to the problem are achievable. One of the first basic steps to visualizing and transforming your life to a happier, healthier state is making time for yourself.

You might be shaking your head over this because I'm sounding crazy right now. That's OK. Setting time aside for ourselves can seem impossible. I know that it can be very hard to find a few minutes to spare, let alone an hour. Even more importantly, the few minutes you find alone are usually spent de-stressing from a toxic situation, working on something that needs to be done, or being interrupted every five minutes by your children or partner.

You may be wondering what "quiet time" is going to do for you anyways. If you find a few minutes to think quietly and more often than not find yourself overwhelmed with lists, schedules, and ideas running through your head. Your internal world is feeling as stressful as your external environment. Is there a way to turn the voice off inside your head? Can you silence the ticking clock? The answer is yes. With these four tips, you will not only be able to enjoy a time of quiet and meditation, but you will pursue intentional reflection that will heal you, guide you, bolster you, and encourage you.

Meditate

You are probably in one of these three groups regarding the art of meditation: in the know, on the fence, or without a clue. Buckle up, we are going to review what meditation is, why you can't live without it, and how to make meditation work for you.

The Art of Meditation

Meditation has been around for a long time, predating formal religions. Although we often link meditation to religious rituals, like yoga or Christian devotions, it involves more than religious practices. Beyond its religious or philosophical origins, meditation means to contemplate something in general. It comes from the Latin word *meditari*, which means to think about something actively. Some examples of this kind of thinking are active planning, practicing, or rehearsing. The idea of active study comes out of the root word *med* which means "to do what you have to do". Therefore, meditation isn't always about emptying your mind or sitting back passively. Meditation is also about reorienting your perspective and awareness. It can be seen as a way to position yourself for transformation and success.

There are many different ways to approach meditation depending on what you need or prefer. For example, some people find using a body scan will give them relief from anxiety or stress and ground them in their bodies. This transfers energy to the self. For others, words of self-affirmation will be helpful when facing self-esteem issues or toxic environments in the home or at work. Whatever the case, there are many kinds of meditation to explore.

One of the first things to consider is the two meditation options: "guided" versus "unguided." Guided meditations are great for beginners who need help learning how to focus. Using a variety of resources—like going to classes or using an app—you will be able to follow the teacher's instructions and learn how to use meditation techniques properly. On the other hand, more experienced practitioners will be able to use silent meditation whether they are following other people's practices and approaches or using their own.

Another choice to consider is "calming" versus "insight." For those who need help coping with stress or anxiety, calming meditations help alleviate distress by diverting attention and energies to positive spaces. While accessing these quiet spaces, you will be able to find peace and work through various coping techniques to keep going on with your day. Insight meditation focuses more on the transformation of the self through positive messages and self-affirmation. This form of meditation is invested in self-identity and personal growth. Many meditation practices, however, combine a little bit of both to provide a more holistic approach to self-care.

Some different types of meditation which I highly encourage you to try include:

Visualization. Close your eyes and picture something or someone. This can be challenging, but it is important to take your time, creating detail until the picture is vivid and clear. Through this process, notice how your mind is working or how your body feels. Reconnect back to the visuals to encourage relaxation.

Body Scanning. Focus on your body. Move from head to toe (or vice versa), noticing the sensations of your body. It might feel like buzzing, tingling, or warmth. Whatever you are feeling, note it and experience it before moving onwards. When you force your attention on your body, you are better able to relax and identify what your body needs at the moment.

Sound Baths. Listen to music. Try gongs, bowls, tuning forks, ambient sounds, or nature sounds. Allow the sound vibrations to draw your attention and focus your mind on a positive image or thought. Music has always been an important aid to destressing, so make sure to try this out when you feel under pressure.

Focusing Attention. This meditation requires a singular focus on breathing. As you breathe in and out, you only focus on your breath. If your mind wanders, gently bring it back to the original breath focus. This calming technique is great for lowering anxiety and stress.

Zen. These ancient Buddhist traditions seek to combine a sense of peace and insight. The focus is, like many meditations, on your breathing. Focus on your stomach and notice the way it moves in and out. Don't try to concentrate on anything else. Through this meditation, you will be able to find alertness and self-awareness.

Mantra. Instead of concentrating on your breath, mantra meditation focuses on a single word, sound, or phrase. Combining this with words of affirmation, you can boost your confidence or compassion, making this a perfect mix of calming and insightful meditation.

Yoga. Yoga meditation techniques bridge the gap between the mind and the body through slow stretching. In various poses, you can increase flexibility, strengthen your neuromuscular systems, and concentrate on your bodily sensations. Through these positions, you are able to relieve tension.

Vipassana. Like more formalized meditations, such as Zen, this kind of meditation is tied to ancient traditions used to examine your life. Within vipassana, you consider your existence and aim to transform completely. This insight-based meditation encourages you to contemplate ideas about human suffering, impermanence, and non-self.

While the idea of meditation seemed easy at first, I learned that keeping myself focused was hard. In our daily life, we are rarely encouraged to detach and consider life, expectations, or goals. Perspective is discouraged because it leads to moderating your impulses, buying less, saving more, and not investing in groupthink. However, there are many other benefits to meditation beyond wisdom.

The Benefits of Meditation

Meditation practices focus on the body and soul, so it is no surprise that these techniques have positive impacts on both. After a few weeks of meditating, I am sure you will notice some changes in your life and mindset.

Physical Improvements. Prolonged stress and the increase of cortisol levels within the body have been proven to damage our bodies. We flood our brains and bodies with an influx of chemicals or cave into bad habits, like smoking or snacking on chips. Meditation offers an alternative. With calming techniques, meditation can help you slow down and relax. This gives your body a break. Some of the short-term benefits of meditation include:

- Lowered blood cortisol and pressure levels
- Slower respiratory rate
- Decreased sweat
- Lowered heart rate
- Improved blood circulation
- Better sleep

Mental Improvements. When our bodies wear down, our mental state won't be much better off. More often than not, lack of proper sleep and food can result in poor concentration, depressive states, and anxiety. If we aren't mentally in a good place, we are less likely to get things done and more likely to return to bad habits that put us in an even worse state. Meditation offers a way to end the vicious cycle. Through insightful techniques, meditation can channel your mental energies to more positive thoughts and beliefs that can in turn empower you to make more positive changes in your life.

Discover these benefits for yourself:

- Improved self-image
- More positive interactions with people
- Increased positivity
- Less stress
- More self-awareness
- Higher ability to concentrate

The Steps to Meditation

Meditation doesn't have to be complicated. There are a few techniques to try out. Let's start with a basic focusing exercise for beginners:

1. Choose a positive emotion or mindset you want to have. Assign it a color.

2. Lie down or sit in a comfortable place.

3. Breathe slowly and deeply. Close your eyes and visualize the color.

4. Hold the color in your thoughts as you breathe.

5. Think about what positive elements it represents.

6. As you inhale, imagine the desired color slowly moving over your body top down. The color is slowly covering all over your body, right down to your fingertips and toes.

7. As the color washes over you, imagine unwanted feelings seep away. As you exhale, replace the feelings with the color and emotion you want to see in yourself.

8. You can work on this visualization technique for as long as you like. Aim for 1 or 2 minutes starting out.

Another common meditation technique is the body scan. This technique is a great way to reconnect with your body to understand what you need physically while simultaneously giving yourself a break.

1. Lie on your back or sit on a comfortable cushion.

2. Close your eyes.

3. Breathe in.

4. As you breathe in and out, focus on the way your body touches the floor or cushion.

5. Start from the top of your head or the bottom of your feet and slowly move up or down over your body, noticing how each part feels. Keep a lookout for pressure, temperature, tingling, buzzing, or tightness.

6. As you pause over each area of your body, take your time to focus and experience the sensation fully before moving to another part.

7. Gently focus your mind back when it wanders.

8. At the end, open your eyes, breathe freely, and take a moment to evaluate your experience before ending the meditation time.

With these easy meditation techniques, I discovered ways to maintain my serenity. Once I learned how to use these breathing techniques, I could use them anywhere, anytime! Whether I was in my car, trying to calm down from a particularly stressful shopping trip, or going to work, I could set aside five minutes and use meditation to find my inner serenity and resolve.

Journal

The idea of sitting down to think things through with a journal sometimes feels like a waste of time to me. I wonder, "Perhaps there is a better way to use my time?" Short answer: no. As the proverb goes: a stitch in time saves nine. Strategizing and scheduling are crucial for long-term, healthy time management. The key is to find what works for you.

The Art of Journaling

Not everyone is a writer. When you journal, you don't have to be. Even if you don't feel great about your penmanship, there are amazing digital alternatives to explore. Sometimes, however, even the most positive kind of journaling techniques, such as bullet journaling, can lose its impact when there is too much focus on visual appeal. Find a balance of self-expression, efficiency, and comfort when it comes to developing your journal style. This is because journaling can actually fill several needs in your life!

Get Organized. With a well-laid-out planner, bullet journal, or time management app, lists and planning need not be a hassle. The key is to understand what you need for organization. Some apps and planners are more focused on long-term important events with little to no space for personal writings or creativity. Once you know what kind of journal you need though, you can get to planning your daily, monthly, and yearly goals as well as make lists and fill in habit trackers.

Explore Emotions. If your journal has space for diary-like entries or has a mood tracker, you will be able to use your journal to explore your emotions and understand your emotional state over longer periods of time. You'll be able to track positive and negative trends in your life which will help you become more aware and gain more perspective on situations that trigger negative emotional states in your life.

Encourage Gratitude and Compassion. Other diary entries can focus on simple positive affirmations that encourage you to look optimistically at your life. Gratitude journals and compassionate self-affirmations towards yourself or others can rewire your brain, training it to explore options and to stand resilient against difficult environments or situations. I find that positive thinking not only uplifts my soul but supports others around me who may also be struggling.

Be Creative. If there are spaces in your journal or planner for creativity, it's a great tool for using art as therapy. You can doodle or sketch one mandala a day without focusing on shapes, just following your instinct. Don't try to make meaningful pictures, but over time, you may begin to be able to interpret your own artistic expression. Leaving room for art or free writing (where you just write what comes into your head) will allow you to process your thoughts and feelings without judgment.

Trace Success. On days I feel down and unmotivated, I sometimes look back at the things that I accomplished in my journal. If your goals are clearly laid out, you are not only able to see what you want to be done, but also what you accomplished over the day, week, or year! It is important to remind yourself that you have been successful in the past and your future can also be filled with accomplishments. With simple goal trackers for drinking water, exercising, or reading books, I'm able to trace the things I've accomplished. It's a great feeling!

Overall, it is easy to see that journaling was another great step for me. For my first bullet journal, I used a simple lined notebook I bought at a dollar store. Over time, I was more invested in bullet journaling. After I proved to myself that I had formed a positive habit, I treated myself to a nice dot grid notebook which I now use every day.

The Benefits of Journaling

There are many reasons why I got into journaling, but the benefits of journaling surprised me in some ways. I knew that I would become more organized. With proper scheduling, I was able to remember appointments, keep on top of due dates, and even set aside time for myself. It wasn't always easy. As I got used to organizing my life, over time I saw small changes in my body and attitude.

Physical Improvements. Thanks to health and fitness trackers, I felt encouraged to set time aside for physical self-care. Whether it was drinking water or setting an appointment to get my body looked at, I began to feel cared for physically. The meditation times I added before journaling set the tone for my planning sessions, helping me to relieve stress and increase my focus.

Mental Improvements. When I journaled, my organization and planning set me on the right path for the day. As a result, I felt more inspired, motivated, and confident moving forward. With periods of self-reflection added, I was able to relieve my stress levels, increase positivity, and jump-start my concentration. Adding free writing or art to your journaling time will help you work through emotions before starting your day.

Sometimes our ideas about what journaling or what diary-writing looks like can hinder us from trying out journaling. For years, I just thought that journaling was like the diaries my grandmother used to fill with her cursive writing. Minimalist bullet journaling and other alternatives since then have changed my mind. Maybe there is a style waiting out there for you as well!

The Steps to Journaling

You might be wondering, "I'm ready to try this journaling thing out. Where to start?" As mentioned above, it's a good idea to think about what you want to do during journaling. This will determine the kind of notebook or planner you will invest in. You may have to experiment a bit to get the style that you need. Below are some journaling formats with accompanying tips on which journaling style would work best with the format.

Daily, Weekly, Monthly, Yearly Planning, and Goal Setting. If you need to get your mind and home space ordered, using a planner or journal for scheduling and goal setting is crucial. You will need space to set goals for short-term (daily and weekly) as well as long-term (monthly and yearly). If your writing is larger, you will want to make sure the size of your planner space is larger for writing.

- ThoughtSpace Journals Store - Yearly, Weekly, Monthly, Daily Planner

- Productivity Planner

- Bullet Journaling

- Any.do (app)

- Google Calendar (app/site)

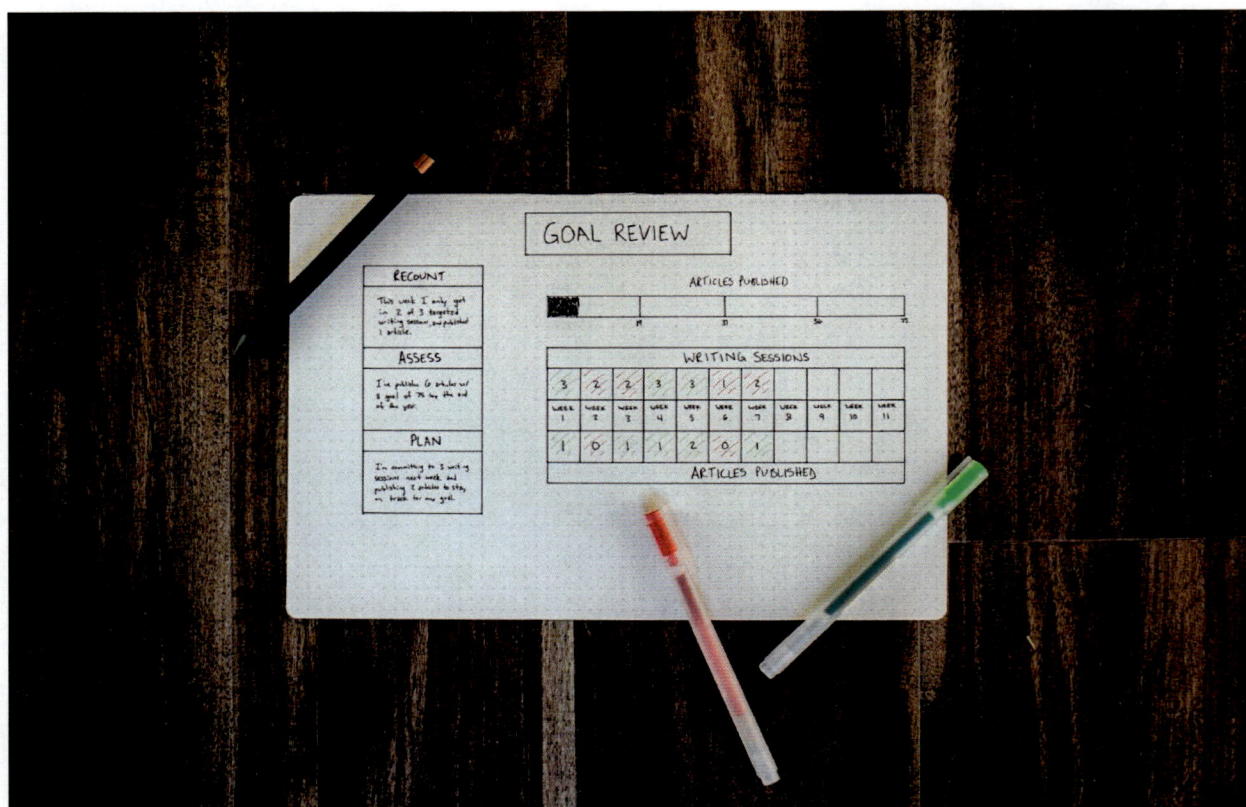

Habit, Mood, and Other Trackers. Do you want to encourage yourself to drink more water, read more books, eat more fruit, or exercise more often? Trackers are a great way to remind yourself to get little things done throughout the day. They can tend to be very limited in scope depending on which journaling notebook or app you use. If you feel like you need some trackers, you may have to use another option on the side along with your preferred notebook:

- The Clear Habit Journal

- Bullet Journaling

- Habitica (app)

- Strides (app)

- SnapHabit (app)

Gratitude Journal. Instead of looking forward into the future, take the time every day to cultivate gratitude. This kind of positive thinking will help propel you forward during more difficult times. Not all planners have space for gratitude or other self-affirmative sentences, you can make the space in journals and notebooks. Every day, write a sentence about something that you are thankful for. It can include a short sentence, a photograph or picture, an achievement, inspirational people or quotes, things you like, or positive coincidences. Read through these moments whenever you are struggling. Your own life is ready to give you perspective:

- The Happiness Project One-Sentence Journal: A Five Year Record

- Good Days Start With Gratitude: A 52 Week Guide To Cultivate An Attitude Of Gratitude

- Bullet Journaling

- The Five Minute Journal App (app)

- Daylio (app)

Creative Journal. Whether you enjoy doodling, sketching, or writing, it is important to get your creative juices flowing first thing in the morning. Journaling can be a great way to guide your creativity, especially with the right notebook. Going for a dual notebook with half-blank pages, half-lined pages is a good start, but other journals can help you target your artistic sensibilities if you want to focus on inspiration. For those who aren't into art, doing something as simple as drawing or coloring in a mandala is an easy way to approach art. With other journals, like bullet journaling, you can make yourself space for free writing or exploring memories:

- 365 Days of Art: A Creative Exercise for Every Day of the Year

- Wreck This Journal: Now in Color

- True You: A Self-Discovery Journal of Prompts and Exercises to Inspire Reflection and Growth

- This Is My Life: A Guided Journal

- Bullet Journaling

- Penzu (app/site)

- Momento (app)

Dream Diary. Keeping a dream diary is a great idea for some. Whether you have the occasional vivid dream or experience lucid dreaming, keeping track of your dreams helps fuel creativity, process emotions, and get perspective on negative situations. Sometimes when we are dreaming, we are subconsciously consolidating memories or situations. Carl Jung, a famous psychologist, believed that dreams may serve as warnings or reveal our psychological struggles to us. Either way, keeping your journal beside your bed with a pen ready is a great way to get started. You will need to have a journal that has dedicated space for writing a dream down quickly:

- Strange Dreams: A Journal

- Dreamer's Journal: An Illustrated Guide to the Subconscious

- Bullet Journaling

- Lucidity (Android app)

- Dream Journal Ultimate (app)

However journaling may look for you, it is a great opportunity to make time for yourself, so that you can assess your goals and situation. With the help of journaling as a form of self-expression and organization combined, you will feel more empowered to chase your dreams and find your happiness!

Breathe

Sometimes my days get so busy, I feel like I don't have time to breathe. Whenever you are feeling swept off your feet and caught in the rush of getting things done, you can start to lose sight of what is truly important and might find yourself derailed from chasing your life goals. I began to realize that there were ways that could help me slow down and, in more emotional situations, help me find equilibrium.

The Art of Breathing Exercises

There are a variety of breathing exercises that you can try out. Not all of them may work for you since some of them require time, space, or certain physical capabilities. I found some to be very simple, requiring around 5 minutes of my time while others might require the privacy of my home and longer periods of time. Here are a few of the popular breathing techniques available to explore!

Deep Breathing. This exercise consists of breathing in the air to the fullest and then fully exhaling, letting all the air out. This style of breathing exercise helps relieve anxiety, brings more oxygen into your blood, and stabilizes your heart rate.

Belly Breathing. With one hand on your chest and one hand on your belly, monitor the movement of your diaphragm and stomach as you breathe. This form of breathing helps you breathe easier and lowers stress. It strengthens your lungs and helps them work more efficiently.

4-7-8 Breathing. This exercise requires you to relax your breath. Breathe in for four seconds, hold your breath for seven, and then exhale for eight seconds. This technique helps reduce anxiety, get you to sleep, or control your temper. I find that it helps me fall asleep, this technique is great for relaxation.

Breath-focus Breathing. It can be hard to stay focused on breathing, so this technique encourages you to think of imagery, words, or phrases to focus on while breathing. The images or words you choose should be positive and encourage you to let go of tension and anxiety while increasing peace and calm.

Lion breathing. Traditionally a yoga practice, this breathing exercise relieves tension in your chest and face. Its focus on stretching your face while breathing in and out can deeply relax muscles within only a few minutes.

In tandem with the meditation techniques I mentioned above, these breathing exercises are a perfect complement and will add physical elements to your meditation. Many breathing exercises add physical boosts to your health and focus.

The Benefits of Breathing Exercises

Studying breathing exercises brought into focus the importance of clean air for me. Until I started to use belly breathing, I had never really given the quality of air in my lungs much thought. However, with increased oxygen, I began to realize that my mental state was changing. I have since come to realize through research and experimentation the ways breathing exercises improve my physical and mental condition.

Physical Improvements. When I take the time to meditate and breathe, I usually feel more alert and energized for the day going forward. Although everyone's bodies and situations are different, trying breathing exercises is a good first step to help your body get the rest and relief it needs. Here are some physical benefits to doing regular breathing exercises:

- Improves blood flow
- Lowers heart rate
- Naturally relieves pain
- Improves posture
- Increases energy
- Relieves muscle tension

Mental Improvements. After a breathing exercise, I usually feel more awake and ready to start my day. Part of this is due to the fact that I have introduced oxygen into my bloodstream, and my brain is now positively responding to the fresh air. All things considered, it is amazing what these short exercises can do for someone's mental health.

- Lowers anxiety

- Increases focus and concentration

- Helps regain perspective

- Reduces anger

- Brings positivity

- Eases symptoms of depression

The Steps to Breathing Exercises

When starting with breathing exercises, it is a good idea to start in your home in a quiet spot where you can relax uninterrupted. Once you are settled and ready, you can try this beginner's breathing exercise!

1. Lie down face up on a comfortable mat or sit on a cushion.

2. Close your eyes.

3. Breathe in naturally.

4. As you breathe in, focus your attention on your breathing. Notice how your stomach and chest move in and out.

5. Keep focused without increasing the rate of breathing. If your mind wanders, gently bring it back.

6. After two minutes, slowly allow yourself to come back to consciousness.

You can try out the 4-7-8 breathing exercise as well! It is recommended to do this no more than twice a day and for beginners to limit yourself to repeating less than four cycles of the exercise during a session.

1. Lie down or sit in a comfortable position.

2. Raise the tip of your tongue so it rests behind your top front teeth.

3. Exhale all the air out of your lungs.

4. Breathe in through your nose quietly for four seconds.

5. Hold your breath for seven seconds.

6. Forcefully exhale through your mouth. As you breathe out, purse your lips and make a whooshing sound for eight seconds.

7. Repeat this up to four times.

Many people underestimate the importance of oxygen in their life. Not only is breathing a way for you to find a quiet space and regain serenity, but it helps physically relax and energize you. Set time aside for breathing exercises, and you will be sure to experience serenity, focus, and positivity!

Affirm

When I first heard about affirmations, I was on the fence. I mean, does saying something to yourself really make things happen? It turned out that I didn't completely understand what affirmations were about. Once I learned the process and the benefits of self-affirmation, I began to use them thoughtfully with my meditation and breathing exercises.

The Art of Self-Affirmations

Affirmations are confident statements made about a truth that you believe or want to realize. As we know, rote learning is a way for us to make something stick in our memory. Since our brain can be rewired through habit, repeating self-affirmations daily can create new neural pathways of positive thought. These changes in our brain will subconsciously encourage us toward a more positive way of thinking. If you feel like your thoughts are more often negative towards yourself, then this strategy will benefit you immensely over time.

Famous psychologists, such as Carl Rogers, believe that our environment and our internalized beliefs about ourselves play an important role in our identity. This is why it is important to be encouraging and supportive about positive life choices for our friends and family. The impact of what we see on social media and TV can also affect the way we view ourselves. Self-affirmation takes these similar events and offers a more positive space for uplifting input.

The best kinds of self-affirmative sentences focus on healthy character traits, such as kindness, openness, integrity, love, or respect. Whatever you choose to focus on, self-affirmations can be written or spoken. Repeat them aloud and think about them during meditation and breathing periods. Write them as inspirational quotes in your journal. In this way, the self-affirmations you have chosen will become a habitual thought that will, over time, affect your behavior and mindset.

The Benefits of Self-Affirmations

Due to its reliance on managing neuroplasticity, self-affirmation has a more positive impact on your mental health than on your physical health. However, when you are mentally feeling, optimistic and energized, you will find yourself able to take better care of yourself in all areas of your life, from achieving goals to your health and fitness. This is because self-affirmation gives you the mental tools to gain a new perspective on yourself and your world, empowering your transformation.

Mental Improvements. Effective affirmations rely on the brain's inability to sometimes tell the difference between reality and imagination. In this way, you are activating your brain's power to support you as you create for yourself a new reality.

- Good character qualities such as kindness, integrity, respect, and love

- Energizes innovation and creativity

- Increases self-esteem

- Encourages positive behavior

- Improves productivity and motivation

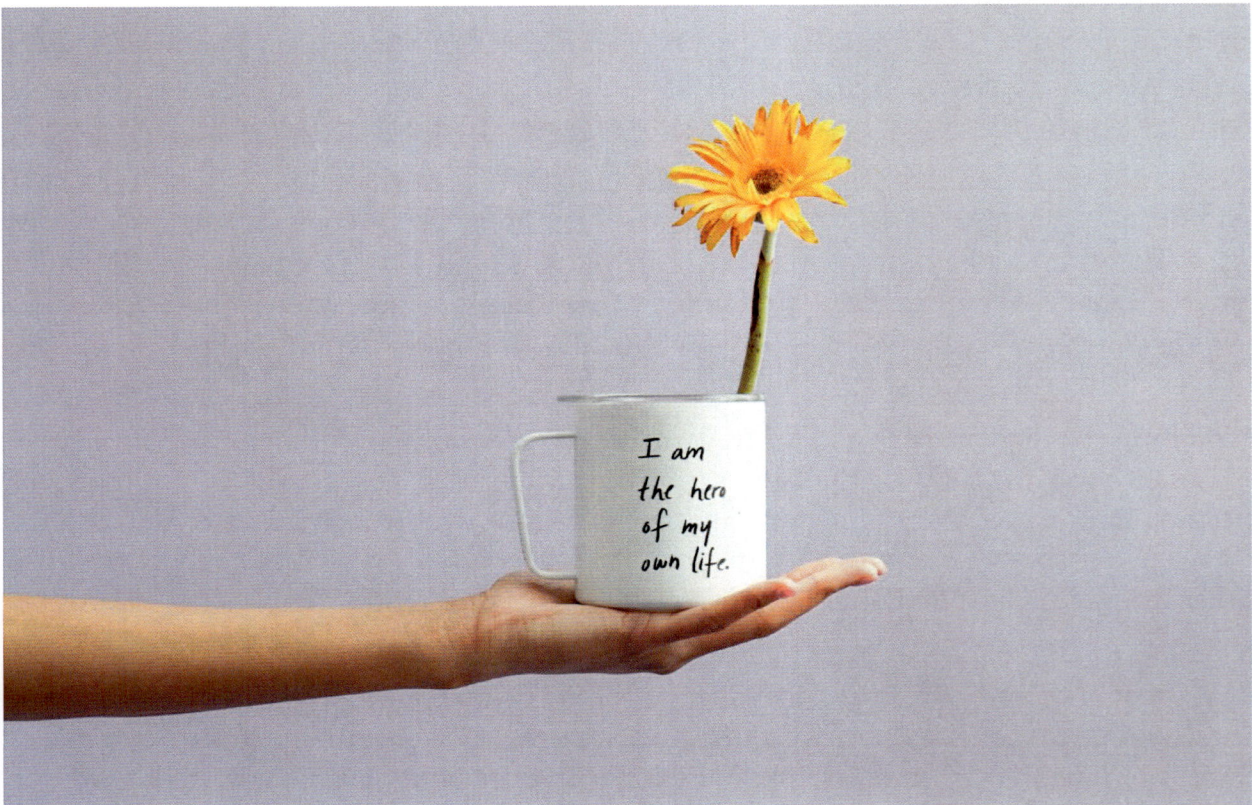

The Steps to Self-Affirmations

When I am meditating, journaling, or doing breathing exercises, I use a short affirmative sentence to think on or repeat aloud to myself. It's more than simply saying, "I am love" or "I can do it." The best affirmations are not rote, but personal. There are a variety of good affirmations out there, but learning how to make your own unique affirmations will boost your confidence and energy in this space.

Write your own affirmation as outlined below. This will provide you with the ability to pinpoint your personal struggles.

1. Think about one thing you want to change right now. Ex. I can't learn all of this new stuff at work. I should just quit.

2. Change the negative situation into a positive situation you want to see. Ex. I want to learn more quickly and become better at my job.

3. Create a word of encouragement based on what you want to see, but write it in present tense verbs. Ex. I am learning many new things at work and overtime will become more comfortable with

4. Keep the affirmation realistic and specific. Ex. I am overcoming the learning curve with the new software at work, and I will feel comfortable with it within two weeks of focus.

5. Link the affirmation to action. Every time you tell yourself your self-affirmation, use it as a prompt to positive action. For example, if you are struggling with new software at your work and are realizing that you are getting too stressed, take a moment to speak the self-affirmation you made and then lead yourself into a breathing exercise, a bio break, or a talk with a coworker.

If you don't feel confident about your ability to tailor affirmations to your liking, you can use inspirational quotes or popular affirmations. Some great affirmations to adopt:

- I possess the creativity for this project.

- Wherever I am working, I am honest and persevering.

- I'm grateful for the job I have.

- My soul is at peace, my mind is open, my body is healthy.

- I am loving, and I share this love with the people in my life.

- These times might be difficult, but they will last for only a short time.

- I am overcoming my illness. I defeat it steadily day by day.

It can be easy to just get down on yourself. More often than not "reality checks" end up being less about keeping yourself grounded and more about giving in to fear or negative self-talk. Self-affirmations are the remedy to fear and negativity, allowing you to step forward with confidence!

Move Forward

The clock may still be ticking. The list of work you need to get through may still be waiting for you. The large variety of stuff to get done before bedtime may still be looming. However, learning to put yourself first is a step towards self-compassion and self-care. As you set time aside for yourself to strategize and meditate, celebrate your achievement. Allow yourself to enjoy a moment of accomplishment and happiness. You have begun transforming already!

Chapter 2:

My Routine

I think we all have that one friend in life who is taking photos on the mountainside of Kilimanjaro or by some waterfall in a South American jungle. Some people have this ability to live life large. So, when someone starts talking about having self-care routines, you might wonder what that might look like for you. Are you a mother and homemaker? Are you a student? Are you deeply involved in your business? Are you facing life as a retiree? Whether you are a tumbling weed or a rock gathering moss, having self-care routines set in place is an important factor to mental health and happiness.

Unfortunately, life has recently made it difficult to stick to a routine. I had a difficult time before Covid-19, but during lockdown, things seemed to amp up. I've seen how it has affected family and friends as well, particularly the uncertainty of lockdowns and opening phases. Some people don't know from one day to the next whether they will be able to work or not. Other people have noticed how their children are struggling with school as they bounce in and out of in-person classes. Covid-19 has also heightened the already stressful atmosphere around shopping. Can I rely on anything these days?

As I pushed my cart down the aisle to find a pack of toilet paper, I realized that the new world I was in was challenging my ability to cope and innovate. I could complain to the store's management. I could start fighting someone for their toilet paper. Or, I could find some alternative way of managing the upheaval of my life.

Throughout the entire situation, I was once again reminded of how important small steps to self-care and routine are for maintaining mental health. Simple choices related to my dietary intake, health, hygiene, and time management determined my energy/self-esteem levels. As I grew my self-respect, self-compassion and recognized my intrinsic value, I started to change my habits and to treat myself better. With each change, I became more confident and motivated, which began a positive cycle of affirmation cycling between better internal and external environments.

I know that we have all been there. It's so easy to get derailed off of a healthy routine, and it's even harder to get back on the wagon! What kind of situation are you looking at right now?

Perhaps you are struggling with a recent move. After settling into your place, you thought that you could return to your previous health and fitness regime, but for some reason, you are struggling to make it happen. You didn't think moving across the country would be a big deal, but somehow it was. With Covid-19 going on, the incentive to get housework done or take a shower has decreased drastically. Somehow you have gotten back into the rut of just not taking care of yourself. Is there a path back to health and wholeness?

On the other hand, maybe you are the person who is obsessed with sharing your life online. You are living for that Instagrammable moment, but recently you notice something is off. The initial joy you had sharing photos has disappeared. More than ever, you are struggling to find inspiration. Behind the scenes of your camera, a world lies in disarray. Is there a way to make your ideal world a reality?

Or perhaps you are that person who struggles with a self-judgemental mindset. Every day, you set a series of goals for yourself and if you fail in one little area, you beat yourself up over it. The result, unfortunately, hasn't led you to success. If anything, you feel worse! You are struggling to sleep at night. You always feel anxious. Sometimes your harshness spills out into your interaction with family, friends, and coworkers, turning you into a strict taskmaster. Can routine include flexibility?

The answer to all of these questions is 'yes'. In many of these cases, revisiting and gaining perspective on routine is crucial. In Chapter One, we began with recharging our batteries, now we need to channel this energy in correct ways to maximize our time and resources. A famous man called Maslow created a hierarchy of needs. In his hierarchy, he theorized that people couldn't just transform themselves into their ideal self without other needs fulfilled. Basic needs like air, water, food, sleep, and clothing are all required for the process of self-actualization. Other needs like stable jobs or good health are necessary as well. This is why we are going to look at setting up routines that get these basic needs covered. I'm going to share some ideas I have about basic routines that will set you up for health and happiness.

Managing Food

It's crazy how automatic reaching for a snack can get. As soon as I plop down on the couch and turn on Netflix, I'm reaching for a bag of chips. At first, I thought that the habit of storing snacks in my kitchen cupboards would stop me. They didn't. Before I knew it, I had formed a new habit of grabbing some water and a chip bag before kicking back in the living room. On really bad days, I'd experience a "snaccident": eating a whole bag of chips in one go. You would think that my weight scale would be enough of a warning signal. It took a while, however, before I realized that I was setting myself up for failure. There were ways I could work around my habits, and part of that included setting up positive reinforcement for the healthier habits that I wanted to form. In the case of managing routines around food, there are a few strategies to consider.

Eat Better, Not Less. It's always a shock when I start trying to change my dietary intake and discover how many approaches result in bite-sized gourmet dishes that barely deal with my stress-eating cravings. In some ways, although many diets are correct in how they portion out meals, it is important to give yourself some room to enjoy healthy snacks, especially when you need it the most.

Plan Meals. . . And Stick to the Plan! As part of journaling, take the time to set up a routine around what meals you will eat and when. For some of us, making time to eat is hard; for others, making an achievable plan and sticking to it is difficult. In the first instance, a good idea is to set aside time on the weekend to make a few meals that will last throughout the week. Preparing a meal that will last two days is another great solution, especially for anyone living on their own. When it comes to challenges surrounding planning meals, it is important to make a list of breakfasts, lunches, dinners, and snacks that you can cook which also have the nutritional values you need. From there, set up a weekly list with enough variety to keep you interested, but with enough ease to make sure you follow the plan. If you are new to meal planning, keeping it simple is crucial for the first few weeks. In order to stick to the meal plan, you can set financial reminders whenever you go over your food budget. Friends and family can also encourage you to keep on target. Of course, the most important way to support positive habits is to make it more beneficial to stick to your plan than not. Make sure you have rewards set in place as well as obvious reminders of how your meal plan is benefiting you.

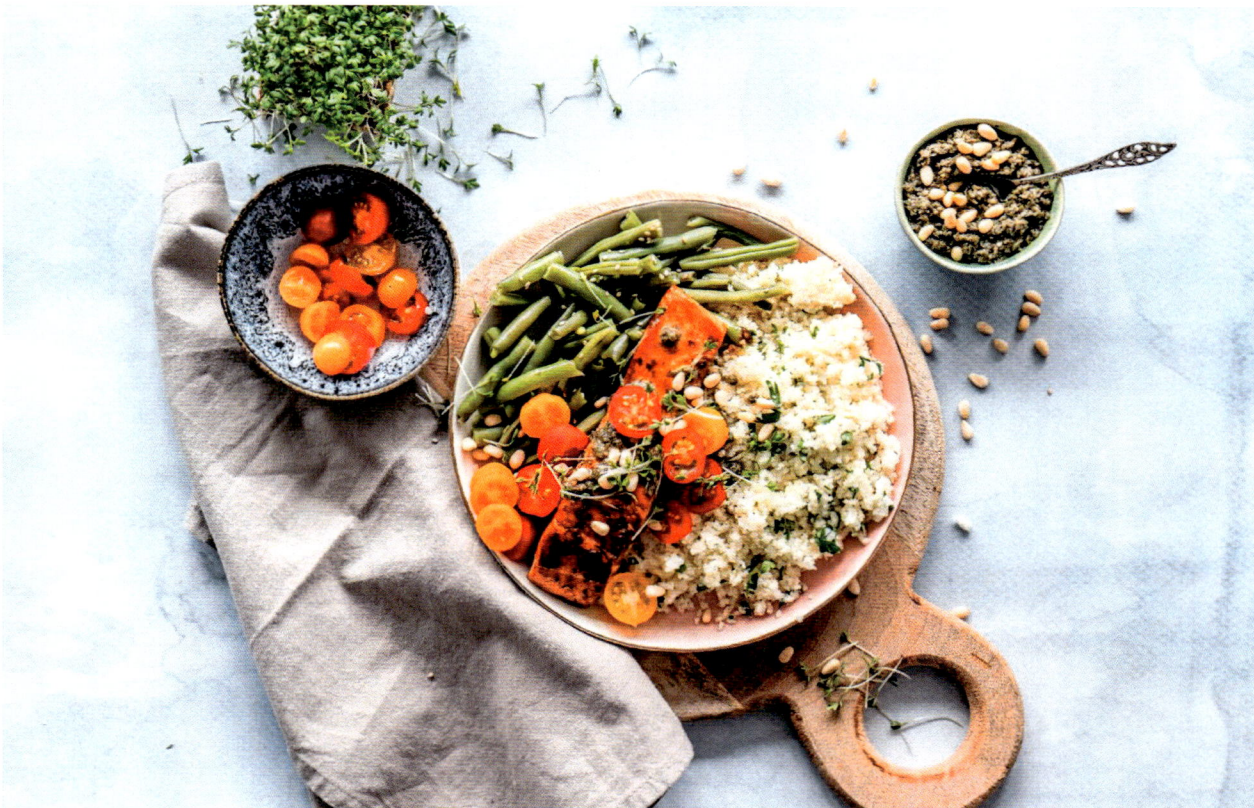

Shop with a List. Walking into a store without a list is probably as bad an idea as shopping while hungry. Both can result in unfocused purchases that may not actually help you make positive choices. Lists are a good way to keep on target, especially if you enjoy wandering up and down the aisles looking for sales. Sometimes you'll see something that you realize at the last minute you need, but for the most part, lists should give you perspective on whether or not you should buy what you think you need.

Find a Partner in Distress. Maybe there is someone in your life who is in the same position as you who needs help when they go shopping. It's a great idea to go together. A supportive partner while shopping can help you gain perspective on impulse buying, encouraging each other to stay on target. Without a doubt, things are always more fun with a friend!

Discuss with your Doctor. You may have realized it's time for a big change. Before you seriously overhaul your dietary intake, a visit with a medical professional such as your doctor, dietician, or nutritionist is always wise. Getting a blood test to check out your insulin or nutrient levels will provide important information on how to move forward. Fitness checks might point you in a different direction, so consulting with a medical professional before taking on a diet is highly recommended.

Dietary Intake

Once you have taken into account your physical needs with professional medical help, you will be able to assess what foods and routines you require for maximum nutrition. You may discover that you need to focus on larger meals at different times of the day, or you might have to graze with smaller portions over the day. Whatever you require, having set times for eating is generally considered healthy for managing insulin levels and stabilizing your metabolism especially.

Diets. Rethinking your dietary habits is a great way to start a new self-care routine. It can be very tempting to just choose a diet that looks yummy or achievable. However, you need to consult with your doctor or dietary specialist first as not all diets will work for you. Some of the healthiest and most popular diets include the following:

- Dash Diet
- Weight Watchers
- The Flexitarian Diet
- Mediterranean Diet
- Mayo Clinic Diet

Healthy Alternatives. Some of you may not need a complete overhaul of your dietary intake. Rather, you could set yourself up for positive choices by replacing less healthy snacks with healthier ones. Reduce the amounts of chips and candy you consume and buy these healthy snack alternatives instead.

- Mixed nuts
- Greek yogurt and berries

- Celery sticks with cream cheese

- Dark chocolate and almonds

- Cucumber slices with hummus

- Hard-Boiled eggs

- Cheese

- Dried, unsweetened coconut

Natural Supplements

Vitamins and herbal remedies are great natural supplements for an energy boost or stress relief. Although you need to be careful about dosage and other medications that may react to your supplements, you can research any side effects easily. I find that Vitamin B complex supplements are particularly important in terms of focus and mood enhancement. Consider these other options for boosting your energy and lowering stress!

- Rhodiola Rosea

- Melatonin

- Creatine

- Vitamin B complex (especially B12)

- Iron

- Beetroot Powder

- Vitamin A

- Vitamin D

- L-theanine

- Vitamin C

- Ashwagandha

- Magnesium

- Lemon Balm

Managing Health and Hygiene

While it is natural to want to have relaxing days spent at home without dressing up, many of us need the support for self-care, through our daily interactions with the world outside of our home. While stuck indoors during Covid-19, quite a few of us may have enjoyed the days spent without worrying about what we looked like. At the same time, many of us felt the lack of motivation seep into our health, fitness, or aesthetic self-care routines. Although pursuing looks for social validation can get dangerous, we need to ensure that we show respect and love for our bodies through our health and fitness choices.

Fitness

Fitness isn't everyone's cup of tea. For some people, just going for a walk around the block is all they can take. On the other hand, there are those people who find running up and down stairs exhilarating. You know who you are. Like your eating habits, your fitness routine needs to reflect your personal physical needs and work with your interests and physical abilities as well. Not everyone can lift weights, but everyone can find their fitness niche, whether it is walking, learning martial arts, or practicing yoga.

With the pandemic in full swing, many gyms were forced to close, which cut off a lot of social and professional support for people who require help when exercising. Classes were canceled, so many have turned to the internet for help, advice, and encouragement. There are a few challenges however when it comes to doing fitness at home.

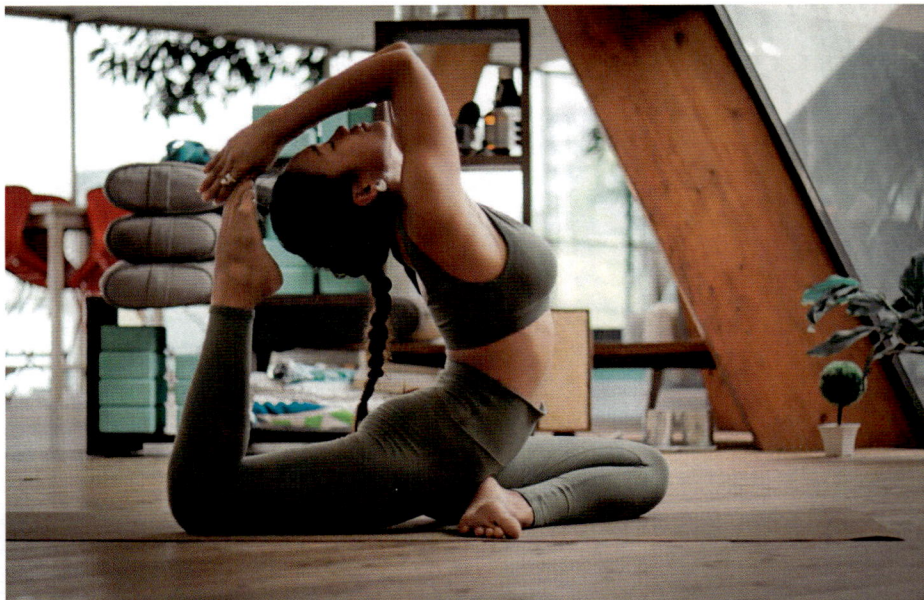

Motivation. If just getting out of bed is difficult, how much harder is it to get into your exercise routine? When your gym is your bedroom, it is challenging to stay motivated and focused. For those who enjoyed their trip to the gym, working out at home might feel impossible. However, while waiting for your favorite gym to open, it is key to continue exercising at least a little bit every day.

Safety. Trained professionals at gyms are great sources of knowledge, not only in terms of instructing how to exercise properly but also how to do so safely. When exercising in your home space, it is crucial to ensure that you have a clear area where you can safely stretch and move about without tripping and falling over.

Motivation and safety concerns should not stop you from forming your own tailored exercise experience at home. With the help of online training professionals, you can form your own workout routines even in limited spaces. Consider the following workout routine for beginners.

Beginner Routine: Each exercise should be done two times with 10-15 repetitions per set and a minute of rest in between.

1. Bicycle Crunch
2. Forearm Plank
3. Stationary Lunge
4. Knee Pushup
5. Chair Squats

If you want more strength-focused routines, you can add dumbbells of varying weights to train muscles. With exercises like push-ups, skipping, dumbbell squats, jumping lunges, and dumbbell calf raises, you will be able to build muscle even when exercising at home.

Cardio Routine: Depending on your level of fitness, each exercise should be done two to three times with 10-15 repetitions per set and a minute of rest in between.

1. Push-ups
2. Skipping
3. Dumbbell Squat
4. Lateral Raise
5. Jumping Lunges
6. Bicep Curl
7. Side Plank
8. Dumbbell Floor Press
9. Crunch
10. Thrusters

If these routines feel overwhelming, don't worry. The good news about fitness is that you can make it work for you! Don't settle for someone else's approach. Instead, explore the many options for exercise, whether it is something like taking the dog out for a walk or biking around the neighborhood. The important thing is to keep moving and find your path to health, fitness, and happiness. The internet has a lot of information on the many ways to exercise and establish fitness routines. Check out these resources and ideas for fitness:

- Get outdoors
  - Jogging around the block
  - Walking in a park
  - Hiking on a trail
  - Biking
  - Getting involved in a sport
- Play active video games
  - Beat Saber
  - Dance Dance 2020
  - Dance Central
  - Ring Fit Adventure
- Watch Fitness YouTube Channels
  - Love, Sweat & Fitness
  - Nick's Strength and Power
  - Joanna Soh
  - HASfit
  - Blogilates
  - Yoga with Adriene
- Use Fitness Apps
  - Jefit
  - Fit Radio
  - MyFitnessPal
  - Find What Feels Good
  - Centr
  - 8fit
  - Fitbit Coach
  - Jillian Michaels Fitness App

Health

With the pandemic ongoing, it seems like now would be the time everyone would be concerned about their health. But I feel like it has become harder to feel heard, especially when there are people around the world who are regularly hospitalized for a serious virus. You begin to think to yourself, "Well, this small problem of mine isn't that big of a deal."

This kind of mentality is made worse by the fact that many of us may be struggling to find adequate health care or proactive medical professionals. Even those who are lucky enough to have a family doctor may still be unable to access services in person. This state of affairs results in many of us not being able to get the help we need. As the world starts to get back on its feet, it is crucial to also get the health support you have been waiting for. In the meantime, there are ways to cope with illness and fatigue, minimizing your health struggles and moving you into a better place where you can make the most out of your life.

Managing Illness. There are a few family and friends in my circle who struggle with chronic illnesses, cancer, diabetes, and COPD (chronic obstructive pulmonary lung disease). Unlike illnesses like the flu or headaches, you don't know if or when you will feel better, so the mental strain during chronic illness can be very high:

1. Eat properly

2. Exercise as much as possible

3. Work through stress with positive activities such as meditation, breathing exercises, hobbies, and exercise

4. Drawing boundaries and saying 'no' to obligations you don't need to do or want to do

5. Building a strong support network with friends and family

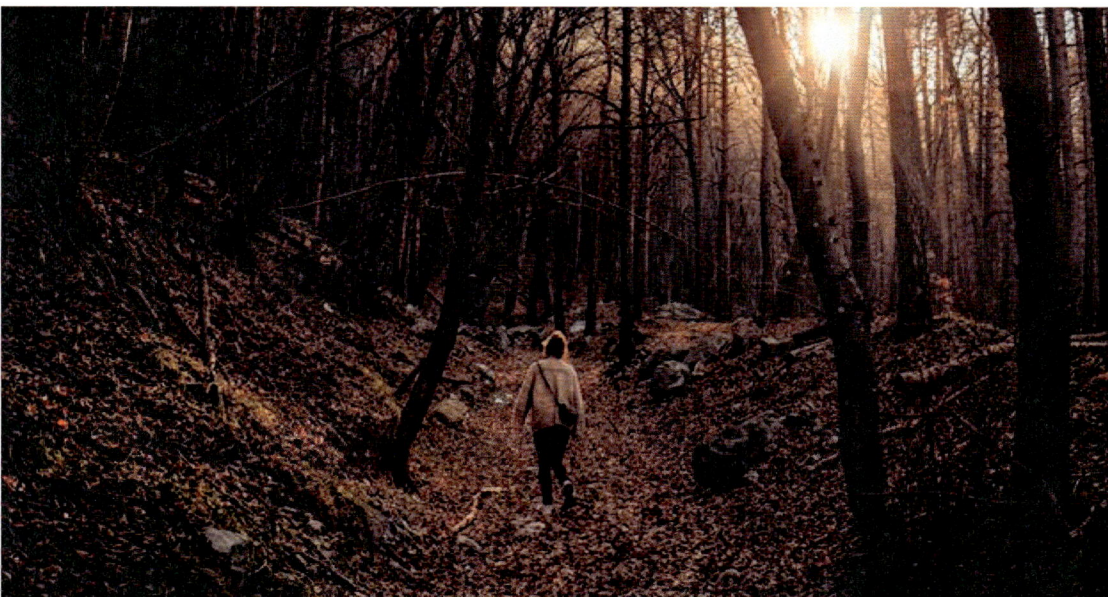

Manage Fatigue. Sometimes part of our lack of motivation and focus is due to fatigue. Feeling tired or listless might be due to physically working too little or too much, struggling to keep a stable sleep routine, ongoing illnesses, or mental health conditions. Depending on the source of your fatigue, your doctor may recommend different treatments. Aside from consulting a professional, there are some other steps you can take to boost your energy and beat fatigue:

- Drink water regularly

- Eat energy-boosting foods like cereal with fruit and yogurt, eggs, oatmeal with raisins, fruit, fish, nuts, and seeds

- Go for a walk or do a few exercise reps

- Cut back on activities in your schedule

- Pursue interests that you love

- Relax with healthy activities such as practicing yoga, making music, or creating art

Taking care of my health is one of the most important ways for me to tell myself that I am valued and important. If I am not able to take care of myself, how am I going to be able to help others in my life? By focusing on my mental and physical health, I am empowered to transform my life and find happiness in even the most challenging of circumstances.

Aesthetic Self-Care

I know the idea of aesthetic self-care is linked to external validation. However, when properly motivated and used as a way to show love and respect for yourself and your body, aesthetic self-care can be an important factor for health and happiness.

Provides Stability. Having a schedule set up every morning after you get up and every night before you go to bed provides a feeling of security because of its regularity. In a world full of panic-inducing headlines, statistics, and news cycles, it can be hard to feel like life is in your hands. However, while the rest of the world might be spiraling out of control, you don't have to be. Maintaining a core self-care routine and basic hygiene standards tells you that you are in control, even in one small area of the world.

Opportunity for Mindfulness. It is all too easy to get into your head, worrying about things that you have no real control over. As mentioned before, this constant flood of anxiety can be overwhelming. By focusing on the sensations of the moment, whether we are scrubbing our feet, enjoying the cool relaxation of a face mask, or taking a bath, we can direct our attention and energies toward taking care of ourselves and listening to our bio-rhythms. Afterward, we may be able to more calmly look at the ongoing situation that had been previously stressing us out with more perspective and self-awareness.

Bonding Moments. Set up a special time and invite a close friend, partner, or family member to spend time with you. Finding ways to hang out, especially as lockdowns ease, can be both encouraging and provide support for a loved one. Through our relationships, we can find joy and contentment even when things around us are less than perfect.

Depending on your priorities and interests, these forms of self-care routines can last anywhere from a few minutes to a couple of hours. For some of you, this might feel like second nature, and you have been able to maintain a healthy schedule of body care habits going. However, for others, lockdown or other life circumstances might encourage them to stay at home and veg at the cost of their health and hygiene. If the latter is true for you, try to make one of these tips a goal for yourself this week.

- Change up your lotions, shampoos, conditioners, and body wash
- Try a sugar scrub or face mask
- Keep a basic hygiene routine going, including shaving, showering, and brushing your teeth
- Set aside a time with a friend to treat yourself to extra attention, whether it is exfoliating, getting your nails done, or getting a haircut at home
- Find ways to keep yourself motivated by making contact with friends and family through videos and photos online
- Curate your wardrobe and treat yourself to a new outfit as a reward

Managing Time

One of the largest obstacles to happiness is poor time management. I'm always surprised by how much I can avoid getting done in a day if I want, but on other occasions, I find myself overworking. It got me thinking about how many times this cycle of inactivity and overactivity stresses me out and pushes me to my limits. Both of them result in anxiety, guilt, and irritation. All of these emotions are especially exacerbated when I go online and see photos of seemingly carefree acquaintances and celebrities living large. They seem to be checking off their bucket lists while I bounce between procrastinating and overworking.

Judging by appearances is a trap that we need to avoid as best as we can, but it is all too easy to play the comparison game. Especially when it feels like we have nothing to show for our efforts. Is there a way to find balance in my life? I believe there is. I began with sitting down and deciding on some long-term goals and strategizing for some short-term goals as well. With the help of journaling and meditation, I was able to focus better and feel more motivated to work toward change. However, I also had to learn how to manage my time better.

While having goals and knowing what you need and want is great, understanding the pace you need for your life is also crucial. For some people, getting three things done in a day is a moment of victory; for others, hopping between activities, events, and job deadlines is the spice of life. Whatever the case, learning how to balance times of activity with times of relaxation and introspection will lead to a more holistic approach to achieving happiness.

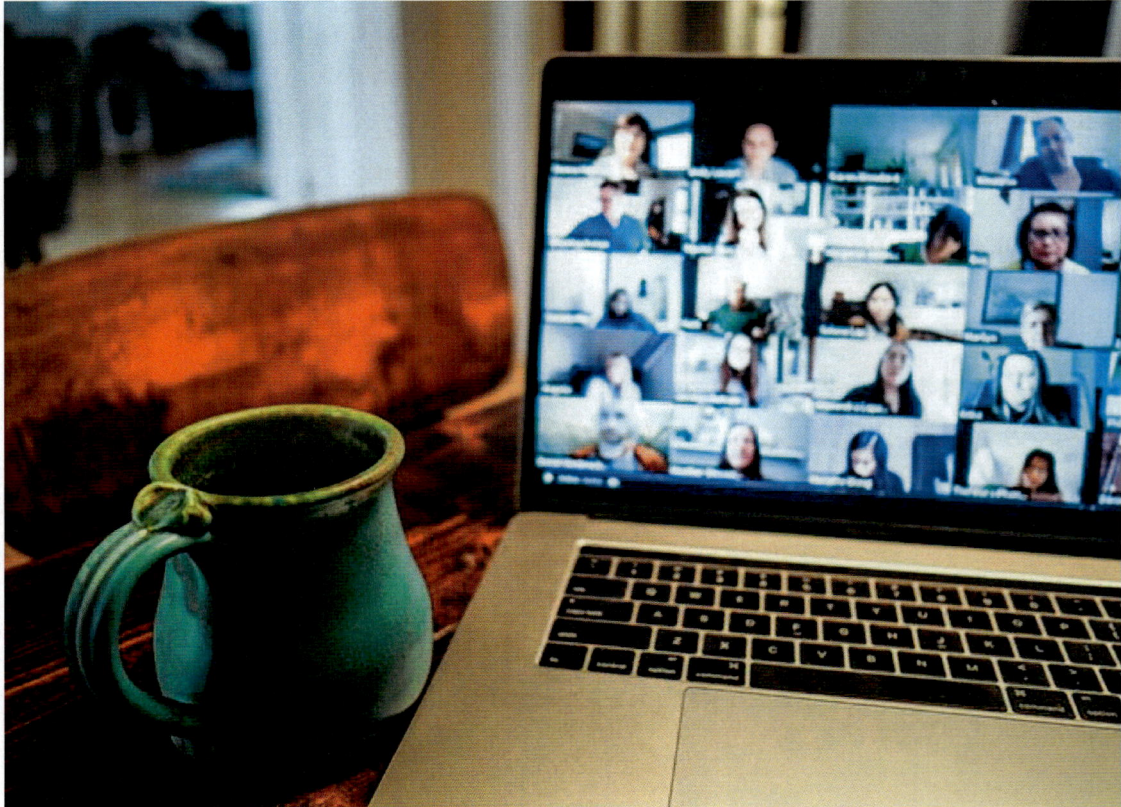

Before deciding what kind of schedule and which routines work for you, you might want to consider some important questions going forward.

- What do I see myself doing in 10 years? How am I living?
- What do I want to accomplish before the end of the year/the end of next year?
- What can I do this month? This week? This day?

Answering these questions in detail might give you some hints as to how to go about work life, home life, and everything else in between.

Balancing Work and Play

"All play and no work makes Jack a dull boy.

All work and no play makes Jack a mere toy."

I remember my mother reading this nursery rhyme to me as a kid. Looking back as an adult, the truth of this children's poetry verse rings louder than ever. Overworked, we lose the whole point of living at all and have no time to enjoy our interests and interact with our loved ones. Without work, we lose the self-determination and self-confidence that comes with achieving goals, maintaining a routine, and challenging ourselves. Somewhere in between is a sweet spot of achievement and relaxation. You might be wondering how to achieve that balance, and a key component has to do with how you view yourself and how you value your time. If you understand that your self-expression is important, you will make sure to prioritize time for you to relax, exercise, and create. However, if you are holding onto subconscious beliefs that your identity and value is tied up with your productivity, you might find it hard to say no to work demands. On the other hand, if you struggle to tear yourself away from Netflix and your couch, you might be underestimating the value of living your own life in creative and productive ways.

In order to get out of the grip of overworking or procrastinating, you may have to go about reorganizing your routines, transforming your mindset about your intrinsic value, or changing your approaches to human interaction. Here are some ways to do that:

- Draw social media and work boundaries by unplugging from your phone for a few hours every night before you go to bed.

- Curate your friendship circles and social media demands, focusing on the important people in your life and muting toxic, negative, or unhelpful friendships.

- Revisit your schedule and minimize the list of activities you have set for yourself or add another goal for you to work on.

- Consider volunteering as a way to keep active without the stress of adding work pressure into your life.

- List the pros and cons of setting boundaries or getting stuff done. Whenever you struggle to say 'no' to work requests or to get off the couch, revisit the list for encouragement.

Working At Home

Pre-pandemic, there were a bunch of people who were working from home already. This was more due to lifestyle choices which may have suited them. At least they were more or less ready to remain home and work. For the rest of us, working from home was a real shock. Many of us had to relearn new boundaries for self-discipline or figure out how to work without the energy of a team. Others had to juggle being a stand-in teacher for their kids. As a result, the boundaries between work and home began to blur in an unhealthy way.

I will admit some of it was my fault. Unlike the extroverts in my family, I wasn't missing the energy and socialization of working with a team. However, sometimes I would find myself getting distracted pursuing interests instead of focusing on my work. When I couldn't get the necessary work done during the day, I would end up forgetting to make dinner as I pushed through my workload late into the evening. Without set habits and proper time allocated to what I really wanted to do, I began to feel stressed out.

To make things worse, some businesses have figured out that they can make remote work positions permanent, removing the need for out-of-home workers to leave their home. I have a feeling that this won't sit well with everyone. Personally, I like the feeling of going away and focusing in an office that isn't in my home, but I have been learning ways to make the most of my stay at home. Recently, I've tried out some tips on how to keep work and life balanced, especially when we are stuck at home.

- Set a schedule for working hours and stick to it as far as you are able
- Create a routine you can follow in the morning to get an "at work" mindset going
- Make sure you have breaks set up for fresh air, eating, or stretching and that you don't cut them short
- Discuss with your partner or roommate, if you have one, about the need for quiet and space while at work
- Set aside, if possible, a separate workspace from your living spaces. If you have a spare room or corner in a quieter nook of your home, set up your workspace there. Don't return there after your set hours are done.
- Keep a separate phone number for work, whether it is a Skype number or a second mobile phone. When you are done working, leave your phone in your workspace if you can.

That covers working at home in general, but what if you have kids running around as well? Usually, with schools opening and closing from month to month, you might find yourself with only a week's notice that your child's holiday will be extended for another three weeks. Since people have different parenting styles, there are two different approaches to coping with working and managing your kids at home.

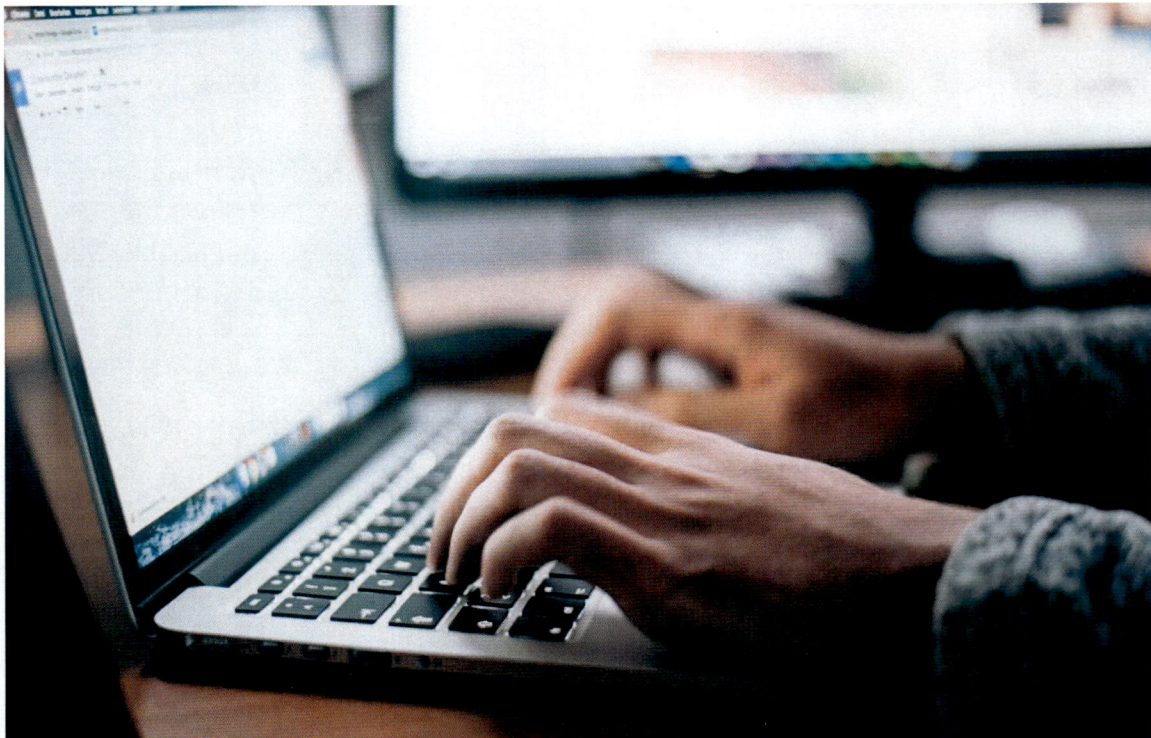

Scheduling. If you prefer to schedule and organize your space, these tips may give you some ideas moving forward on how to negotiate the needs of your work and your children.

- Schedule definitive times for study, play, and eating, which you will oversee for a week and then slowly stop monitoring so you can focus on your own tasks.

- Set a nap or quiet time in the afternoon where your children will be encouraged to stay in their room playing quietly or napping.

- Make a personal workspace for yourself, whether a spare bedroom or closet you can sit in.

- Invest in online childcare or tutors.

- Plan for ways to avoid interruptions, such as leaving the children in the care of your partner, locking your door, or putting on headphones.

Free-flowing. If you don't mind your kids playing on their own, these tips will help you make the most of your time so that you are still able to get some work done.

- Create a schedule with your children and get them invested in following their own routines.

- Create large periods of time where your children go away to play by themselves in predetermined areas of the house.

- Make a working space in the command center of your home so that you can keep a finger on your home's pulse.

- Reward your child with quality time, setting aside special experiences and playdates with a parent.

- Plan for ways to work through interruptions, such as creating nonverbal cues (red ribbons on a doorknob) for times you cannot be interrupted.

Other potential strategies include getting up before your children to get crucial work done, making meals ahead of time, prepping snack and drinking stations, or getting help from family members over video calls.

Healthy Approaches to Hobbies and Interests

Getting involved in creative arts or skilled crafting might seem crazy after a long day of work hassling with kids, coworkers, and—let's face it—your partner. However, investing even half an hour in an interest or hobby of your own is sure to help you discover inspiration, energy, and a sense of accomplishment. Hobbies and skilled crafting require long-term time investment and energy, but the benefits of learning a craft are surprisingly high in number. Even if you feel like you are unable to support a hobby, pursue an interest, do research, or read, it is just as helpful. In any case, you are engaging in new ways to express yourself and your emotions. That's a good thing.

Even if you are ready to start a hobby, it can be a bit daunting to figure out what you should start working on. In Chapter 5, I will share with you the many ways you can use the creative arts to express yourself and explore your feelings. I will also give some tips on how to find a hobby that interests you, where to make connections for exploring your interests, and a variety of lists that can jump-start your creative exploration. The key takeaway in terms of balancing your schedule is that hobbies provide a great way to redirect your energies and allow you to destress after a long day of hard work!

It's Your Life

Let's be honest. We have all been here, getting caught up in the craziness of life. I'm no different. I've gotten caught up in the rat race, especially since I began to work at home. As soon as I find a breather, I wonder to myself, "Why am I here again?" More often than not, I end up losing sight of what I want to see in my life—my dreams, my goals, my happiness. At some point, things reached the breaking point.

That's when I began to sit down and reassess my life and what I was working toward. Instead of just meandering from one thing to the next, I decided to hone my strengths and focus on the things in life that bring me true satisfaction and happiness. Learning to establish myself wasn't easy, but with routines that fit my needs set in place, I was more empowered to engage in the activities, interests, and necessities that bring joy into my life. It's time for you to take charge and make the routines of life work for you!

Chapter 3

My Community

"Can you hear me now?" A pause. "How about now? Can you hear me?"

My mother's text lights up my screen, "I can't hear you!!!"

This feels like a common occurrence these days. As we connect online with loved ones and coworkers, we realize that many people are still unfamiliar with how to handle technology disruptions and difficulties. It doesn't make for the greatest online hangout time; especially with my older friends.

Even if you manage to get into a good habit of connecting with friends and family, you might still find the whole process unnatural or awkward which may cause you social anxiety. When it comes to room chats, you might find that some people are quieter than others. Others are always talking over people, and there is no real way to take them aside and get in touch with them right then and there. At some point, you might find yourself wishing hanging out could be as simple as it was before.

All of this comes at a time when we need a healthy, encouraging community the most. In a world that feels so chaotic and uncertain, spending quiet, intimate times with our loved ones feels more necessary than ever. More often than not, our connection to the past lies within family relationships. Unfortunately, checking in with older family members and friends isn't easy.

I remember one moment, during the Covid pandemic when I was passing by my neighborhood hospital. Outside by the large open windows of the lobby, a family had gathered. The mom had a phone in her hand. Behind the glass, an elderly relative sat in a wheelchair with a nurse at her elbow holding a tablet. It was a strange scene, but also very heartwarming, I thought.

"Isn't that so sad?" A woman who had also slowed down to watch the scene shook her head. Her eyes were tearing up. "It's. . . just. . ."

"It's sad," I agreed, sympathetically. "But with the help of technology, they can still meet. That's pretty nice, right?"

It's not difficult to be pessimistic about the changes we are seeing in the way people relate nowadays. Even without the pandemic, it's becoming harder to be authentic, to share your feelings, to post online. You may feel that your moderate voice is being swallowed by one crowd of opinions or another. I know that I had to take a break from social media because I began to face some tough questions. Who actually cares about me? Who should have input in my life? Whose voices matter?

The more I thought about these questions, the more I began to realize that my online connections weren't providing me with the meaningful intimacy that I needed. I was just wasting my time scrolling through Facebook or Instagram to chuckle over a meme, watch a funny or inspirational video, and generally feel FOMO whenever I saw someone else's "perfect" life. I knew that there had to be a better way to use my time online.

Embracing Intimacy

What is intimacy? Why is it always mentioned when talking about relationships? Well, the word "intimacy" is linked to the word "intimate", which relates to a close friendship over a long period of time. It usually means that the relationship is friendly, warm, and private. However, this personal relationship is not necessarily only found between sexual partners. Intimacy can exist between platonic friends as well. According to therapists and psychologists, of the four types of intimacy, only one involves touching.

Physical intimacy encourages closeness and connection through hugging, massages, kissing, or sexual touching. Mental intimacy involves sharing your interests and values through meaningful conversation. Emotional intimacy is stimulated by showing interest in each other's feelings and caring for each other. Finally, spiritual intimacy requires respect for the other person's beliefs and sometimes may involve shared purpose and values.

Making Room for Intimacy

Unfortunately, intimacy can't just happen. It requires trust, acceptance, honesty, and love. All of these emotions must also be shared through open and authentic communication. It isn't achieved through a thumbs up or a short tweet, but through long, sometimes difficult conversations. How can you turn your home into a space where intentional, intimate relationships can be encouraged?

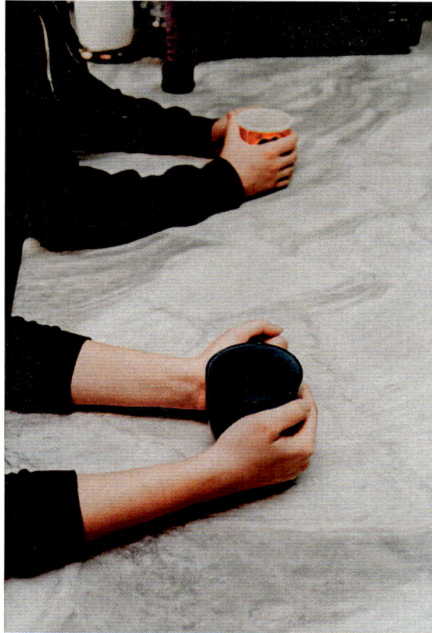

Honesty. Pursuing positivity can be complicated by the desire to look good or to stay in control of other people. Although celebrating the good things in life is a great way to keep feeling inspired and energized, many times the presentation of your home or yourself becomes less than honest.

I was particularly challenged by this when I began to realize that the photographs of my friends were more often less authentic than I thought. The feelings of inadequacy and FOMO I was struggling with were based on misconceptions about reality.

With honesty, I was able to not just share my triumphs but also my struggles. Showing the days that my home was less than perfect, revealing the times I was struggling with a bad hair day, or admitting to ongoing anxieties and conflicts in my life. It wasn't about making drama or stirring up gossip, but about sharing these moments with the people who mattered in my life as a way to authentically connect.

When connecting with loved ones:

- Check-in regularly for weekly updates.

- Remember to ask how it is going and ask for details.

- Be honest about how you feel about a situation.

- Share candid moments of your life without making dramatic statements.

Patience. Building a solid relationship with someone takes time and understanding. Both require patience. Sometimes, you just want to arrive there. After all, it's so easy to get in a car and go anywhere you like. It's so easy to hop onto Amazon and get what you need the next day. It's so easy to surf online and find the information you need right away. The convenience of your life creates expectations that what you want should be able to happen right now, but relationships don't work that way. The people you love and respect are bound to drive you crazy at some point. You are going to struggle with remembering why you want them around. This gets even worse when you feel trapped in a house with them or when you are unable to connect with them meaningfully online.

I began to realize that setting time aside in my schedule to contact one person every other day in a personal kind of way was important. It just wasn't enough to comment on their photo or pop an emoji on their meme. My relationships needed more than that. Although I hated phone calls, I had to phone a few friends once a week. Others, I sent long voice chats to on their preferred messaging platform. Exchanging voice messages turned out to be a great way to connect with many of my friends. For others, video calls were necessary, particularly for my mother.

To be honest, I wish I could say that it was easy. Connecting with my family through video calls often became a chore. Character traits and behavior that annoyed me before multiplied when we hung out online, but sticking through those times paid off. We discovered that we were struggling with similar discouraging situations. We were able to encourage each other and give each other advice. None of this would have happened if I had given up.

When connecting with loved ones:

- Set aside a good chunk of time to connect. Don't expect to meaningfully relate within a few minutes.

- Think twice or countdown before you respond to something annoying or negative.

- Give loved one's space to process conflicts or difficulties.

- Look at yourself through their eyes. From this perspective, you may be able to reconsider your words or behavior.

Respect. People often say that love shouldn't come with strings attached. It's interesting though how respect, more often than not, does. Respect has to be earned, apparently. It gets you thinking. What is respect really about? While you may agree that we need to respect everyone as a human being, there is a feeling that basic social and moral requirements need to be met before you gain respect. This is how society usually discourages negative or toxic behavior. At the same time, you need to recognize the difference between negative behavior and stuff you just don't like.

It reminds me of a former coworker. His personality and self-expression were just jarring to me—his behavior and appearance, mostly. How challenging it was to respect his life and point of view! He wasn't doing anything wrong, nor was he a bad worker. It was up to me to learn how to be flexible and respectful. As I worked through my emotions, I realized that the opportunity for mutual respect had been blocked by my fear of the unknown.

Moving forward with my intimate relationships, I learned that I won't agree with everyone's choices. Sometimes for good reason, too! However, that doesn't mean I can stop respecting them and take away their intrinsic value as human beings. Just like I am prone to mistakes and correction, so too are others in my life!

When connecting with loved ones. . .

- Practice empathy, whether emotional or cognitive. Imagine yourself in their shoes.

- List the positive qualities of your loved ones.

- Create a gratitude list for the role of your loved ones in your life.

- Mature your sense of self-respect. More often than not, when we don't respect ourselves, we will also be harsh and hold unrealistic expectations for others as well.

Love. A lot has been said and written about love. There are definitely many different kinds of love, such as familial or romantic. Passion, desires, and drives motivate you, but love defines the way that you negotiate your bonds between friends and family. Like respect, it can be hard not to attach strings to love. You might find yourself wondering why you still have a certain person in your life. There are moments where you struggle with hating someone because they hurt or disappointed you. Unconditional love holds the key to meaningful, long-term relationships. Learning to confront and forgive people in your life will bring about healthy bonds that can greatly enhance the quality of your life.

Of course, how people can show their love will look different from person to person. That's a fact that comes with its own struggles. It's something I struggle with a lot. How many times have I been annoyed by someone's gift or words of encouragement, only to realize that it was their way of showing support. Sure, it would be nice if people could support you in ways that felt meaningful to you, but not everyone is going to be able to do that.

That's why working on patience in tandem with love helps. I am slowly recognizing that by building meaningful, loving relationships, I have the support and care that I need to get through the challenges I face in my life. Stopping to acknowledge the many ways people have shown love and care for me gives me the energy and motivation to keep going.

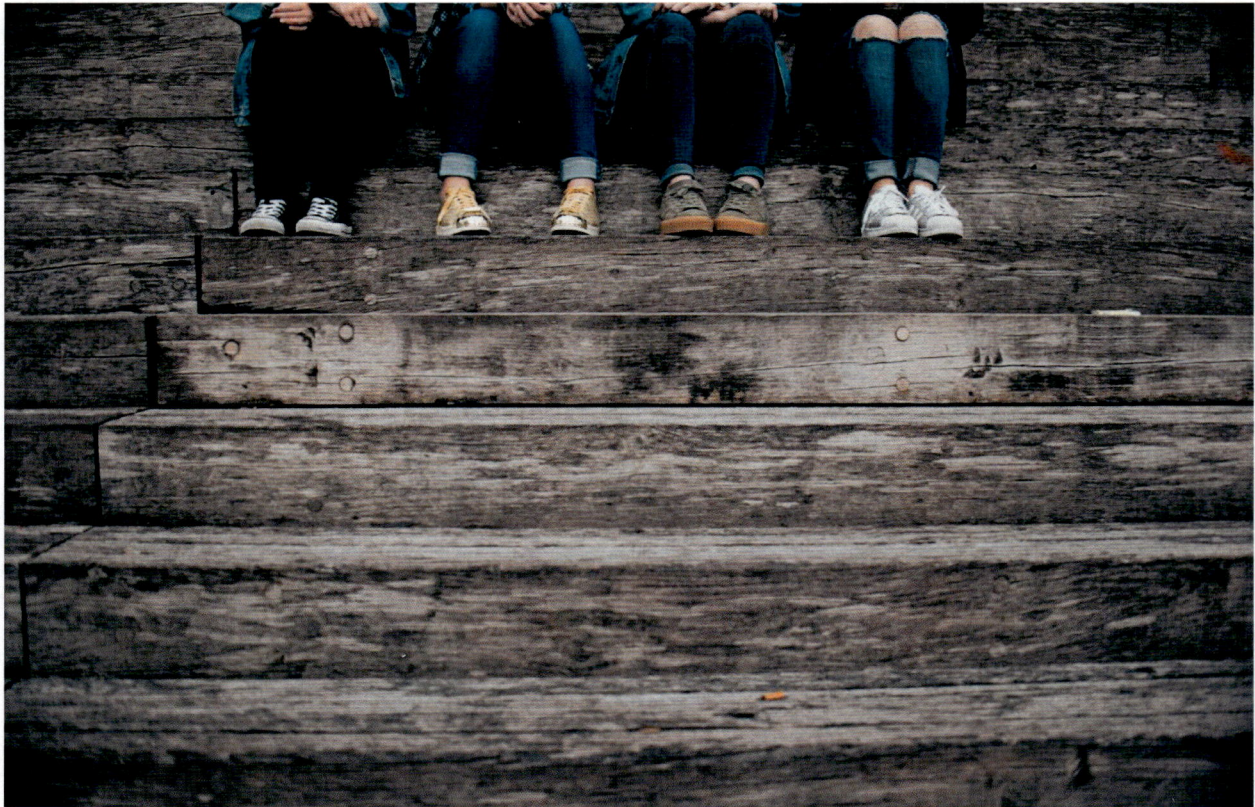

When connecting with loved ones, work toward compromise and understanding. Aim to thoroughly deal with the issue so that there isn't any room for grudges.

Study your own and your loved one's "love languages". Love languages include:

- Words of Affirmation: showing care and affection through words like, "Thank you for. . ." or "You look great!"

- Gifts: giving thoughtful, not necessarily expensive or big, gifts

- Acts of Service: doing something to help your loved one, like finishing housework

- Quality Time: spending time doing something together, like making dinner or going for a walk

- Physical Touch: hugging, holding hands, back scratches, or other physical/sexual touching

Life with Intimacy

When you pursue friendships intentionally, it's more than just having a good time together. It's about encouraging and helping each other as you mature and transform over time. The best kind of relationship builds you up so that you can become the person you are meant to be, achieve the dreams that you have always had, and overcome the challenges that arise in your way. Instead of settling for the Like button or a short tweet, go for true connection and you will begin to reap the benefits of deep friendship.

Lower Your Stress. When you have a friend who actively listens to you and gives you positive input into your life, you will experience less stress. No longer feeling alone and overwhelmed, you might feel like you have backup, whatever happens. You can also in turn provide the same back to them. This interchange relieves pressure, which can also lead to better health.

Prolong Life. With lowered stress, you are less likely to exacerbate chronic conditions or encourage illness. Prolonged stress can cause insomnia, a weak immune system, digestive or heart problems, and high blood pressure. With strong community support, the effects of anxiety, stress, depression, and irritability will ease, allowing you to maintain your health and prolong your life. Intimacy and friendship can in fact extend your life up to 8 years!

No Longer Lonely. Strong friendships in your life can ease loneliness, especially when you are single or childless. Community through intentional relationships can ease social isolation, which results in better mental health. An important factor is having a confidant: a person with whom you can trust your secrets. Having one or two of these people in your life will boost your sense of self-esteem, self-confidence, and self-compassion.

Support for Success. If your physical and mental health are in a better place, you are more empowered to achieve success in other areas of your life. It is all too easy to listen to negative self-talk and toxic input from certain voices in our lives. Reality checks can demotivate us and cause us to question ourselves. Having a second opinion and alternative perspectives can be the encouragement we need to succeed. For some of us, we need friends to let us know that we can do it. For others, we need to be grounded in reality and understand what we can actually achieve. Friends can push us, but they can also let us know that it's OK to relax.

As a result, to miss out on intimate, intentional friendships is to miss out on support and success in life. Intimacy provides us with perspective because it involves loving input as well as thoughtful listening. It isn't about talking about the weather or engaging in small talk about shared interests. This kind of long-term relationship relies on being honest about your struggles and emotions beyond the daily grind of life. I am thankful for the few people in my life who have become my core group. It's time you too find your own intimate circle!

Circles of Friendship

While looking at your Facebook friend lists, you might be thinking, "Well, I have a lot of friends on my Facebook, so I'm good, right?" Right? Well, maybe not. After all, quantity doesn't equal quality. The reality is that it is a rare person who can equally give themselves to more than a handful of people at a time. At some point, there is going to be neglect somewhere. This is why the kinds of relationships you are experiencing can not be understood in terms of numbers alone.

As soon as I realized that my energy was being diverted into potentially less than helpful areas of my life, I began to rethink my Facebook friend list. As I scrolled through the names, I knew whom I could "unfriend" fairly easily. I didn't though. After all, removing Facebook from your life entirely doesn't mean that you will become instantly happy. Sure, it might relieve some stress or decrease negative input, but the reality is that our plugged-in world does require some social networking and a wide variety of acquaintances.

On the other hand, it is important to put these kinds of numbers and relationships in perspective. Acquaintances, even the nicest of them, are not going to be able to provide you meaningful emotional support. The odd "I'm rooting for you!" feels nice but ultimately unhelpful. Think about the "thoughts and prayers" tweets that happen after every natural disaster or tragic incident around the world. While the emotions may be authentic and the responses supportive, they are more meaningful when they come from people who are actively participating in your life and giving you practical support for your transformation and happiness.

I didn't deactivate my social media accounts, but I began to rethink how and why I was using them. I began to sit down and think about what I was looking for and where I could actually get what I needed. It took some time and introspection, but after a while, I began to realize that if I was to find happiness in the 2020s, I would need to curate my friends and focus on just a handful of them. Not only would I gain the support and encouragement I needed moving forward, but I would also be able to give equally back.

Analyze

How am I going to figure out who should be in my intimate friend circle? Well, for those who are married or have kids (or both), the obvious answer is your partner and your children. Beyond that, who else? Do your parents automatically count as intimate? Which friends online would make the cut? In order to help you figure out who is a candidate for meaningful investment, consider the following questions:

- Who has contacted me with a question about my life in the past 72 hours?
- Who asks me detailed or leading questions about situations I am going through?
- Who is likely to find ways to help me practically at any time of the week?
- Who seeks out my help, advice, or input in return?
- With whom have I fought and made up?
- Who has been around the longest and interacted with me the most?

From these questions, you may figure out that you have a couple of friends or more. If you end up with only one or two, don't panic. Life may have something for you around the corner! If you discover that beyond your partner, you don't have any intimate relationships, this might be a time to start looking for an alternative voice in your life.

Whatever the case, take the time to think over these relationships, recognizing the good times and the bad. Embrace gratitude for what you have been given. Begin to consider ways to maximize time and resources for these important people. They deserve your attention and care!

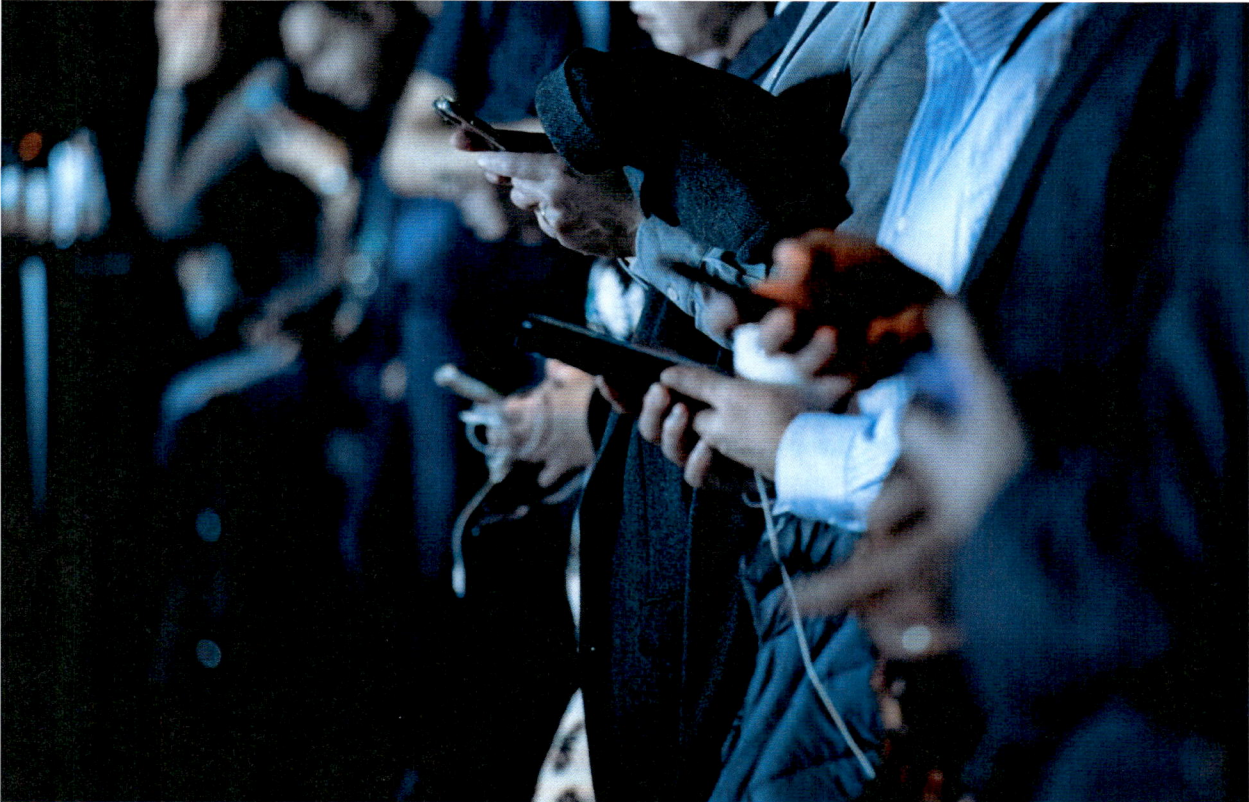

Minimize

In tandem with moving toward intimacy, this period of change holds a call to transform your communication habits in person and online. It's time to make social media work FOR you, instead of running around and trying to serve the faceless mob. Maximize the networking opportunities for career and personal life by tweaking your social media feeds. In doing so, you will be able to choose whom to pay attention to and whom you can ignore.

- Get out of and remove toxic relationships from your life.
- Mute your phone after 6 PM.
- Uninstall social media apps for a week or so just to take some time off.
- Keep your phone on during work hours only.
- Turn off social media notifications, so that you control the apps and the apps don't control you

With a minimized and controlled social media, you will rediscover time and energy to talk with the people who are important to you. You will no longer get distracted by the world at large, overwhelmed by unhelpful debate, or depressed by the illusions of FOMO. You will discover where happiness truly lies in meaningful, day-to-day interactions.

As you relegate social media to a role used as a tool for communication, you will discover the importance of keeping your work and home life separate. By keeping your interactions with acquaintances limited to work hours, generally speaking, you will be able to reclaim hours in the evening for creative expression, uplifting activities, and intimate community.

Socialize

As stated in the previous section "Embracing Intimacy", you can leverage the positive qualities of honesty, respect, patience, and love to sustain intimate social activity and a supportive community. This doesn't mean that you have to throw social media out of the window entirely.

I realized that my instinctive backlash to social media—to just remove it—wasn't helpful. So I learned how to focus on responding meaningfully to posts that my friends made instead. I began to rethink what I was sharing online as well. In this way, I was able to find authentic encouragement and practical support which I could reciprocate.

- Ask yourself before posting a response: what does this friend need?
- In private, contact struggling loved ones and offer practical support.
- Review what you post online before you post it. Ask yourself: what does this post say about me? Does it increase my sense of identity or happiness?
- Every few days, check-in with a friend privately to see how they are doing.

Your situation, your life, and your friends will require unique approaches that will only work for you. As the world slowly leaves their homes to reacquaint themselves with their neighborhoods and communities, you will be given a fresh opportunity to build firm foundations with your friends and family. Whatever the situation, I firmly believe that if you invest time and energy into the people who actually care for and about you, your path to happiness will be made easier.

Alone Time

If intimate relationships play an important part in mental health, supportive networks, and long-term happiness, is spending time alone such a great idea? Actually, yes! That's because your quiet time is in fact another sort of communion. It is an opportunity for you to dialogue with yourself, stepping back and listening to what you are thinking and feeling.

I know that this sounds crazy. It is always jarring to hear people talk to themselves out loud when you least expect it, but the fact is that it is beneficial for everyone to carry on a mental or verbal dialogue with themselves. These conversations can play many different kinds of roles. They can be reminders, self-affirmations, encouragements, or even questions. Here are some ways to learn how to listen to yourself.

- Use mood tracking apps or journal modules.

- Keep a small journal with you as you go through your day and take note of your emotions and thoughts. What are you telling yourself? Is it mostly positive or negative? What events lead to these thoughts? How did negative self-talk hold you back? How did positive self-talk help you?

- Visualize a witness stand and interrogate the negative self-talk you thought of or heard. How much of it is true? How accurate is it? Is it a fact or opinion? How big of a deal is it really?

- Transform the words into self-affirmations.

- Create a positive mood board collage. Using magazines, newspapers, etc, create a collage of keywords, phrases, or pictures that represent the most positive aspects about yourself and your life.

- Look back at your life experiences and find the memories that push back against the negative self-talk. If you are feeling like you never succeed, for example, go back and think of a time when you did succeed at something, even if it wasn't something very big.

How you engage in dialogue with yourself is determined by your own needs, but you can be certain that stepping back and looking at yourself, known as self-awareness, is a good step toward better mental health and happiness. By looking at yourself and listening to your intuitions, you are better able to know what you want and need. Instead of being pushed and pulled around by less than helpful input from the outside world, you will be able to pursue meaningful connections, get practical help, and find happiness within your relationships.

Chapter 4:

My Home

Every now and then I hear someone talking about how much they got into home renovations during Covid-19. Some of my friends seem to have taken the opportunity to get some much-needed home decor going. Others wanted to redecorate or get some spring cleaning done. I'm suddenly sitting there, thinking, "Should I be changing things up at home as well?"

Looking around, I had to admit, something needed to change. I hadn't gone full hoarder, but the level of unnecessary stuff and trash in my home was nearing critical mass. You have probably experienced many different kinds of living spaces in your life. There are the Comfy Hoarder, the Garbage Collector, and the Catalog Spaces. Each one represents a different kind of person. Although it might be easy to point at one kind of home space and point the finger at the glaring problems, other approaches have their own pros and cons.

Take the Comfy Hoarders. When you walk into their front hall, you are greeted with shoes, coats, piles of bags, and shopping items still in their bags. The disorganization continues into the living spaces, but you don't mind. It's clear that a family lives in this house from the arts and crafts littering the dining room table to the half-opened pantry spilling out snacks. It isn't a terrible place to hang out. It feels kind of inviting and homey because you feel like everyone in any state of mind is welcome here. There is a warm authenticity about the place. The only problem is that you put your keys down somewhere and you can't find them again. It makes you wonder, "Could my home be comfy AND organized?"

Then there are the Garbage Collectors. They might not be living in the largest homes or apartments, and they might not even own many pieces of furniture or things. However, when you step through the door, you are confronted by rows of recycling not yet taken out. Perhaps full garbage bags are hanging about. Boxes with stuff "to go to charity" are not yet taken out. Any flat surface is covered with pop cans, chip bags, and other trash that need to find a home in the dumpster. Underneath all the mess, you can see that the place is nice but that huge chunk of trash has to go! A few hours of scrubbing wouldn't hurt the place, either. You ask yourself, "Would a little bit of self-discipline make my home more hospitable and inviting?"

Finally, the Catalog Spaces. These homes are the most daunting to enter because you realize that perfection does indeed exist out there. As if they were taken out of an Ikea catalog, these homes not only sparkle, but they have an air of sophistication that makes you question your ideas of home decor. Everything seems so matchy-matchy and color-coordinated, you begin to wonder where the personality of your friend went. The walls are full of high-quality art and photography, but something seems to be missing. You can't put your finger on it though. So instead, you find yourself saying nice things about a home that could very well be a hotel room. When you return home, you might struggle a little with feeling inadequate, but you also wonder, "Can my home express my interests and taste as well as be beautiful?"

The answer to all of these questions is a resounding "Yes!" The truth is that our home spaces can be organized, tidy, and clean without losing our sense of self. A little bit of self-discipline and organization goes a long way, but this is all supported by an awareness of what we want from life. If we aren't pursuing intentional living, then our home spaces will also reflect the disorganized life we are leading.

In the end, your home is just a tool to empower you, creating a sanctuary for relaxation and a safe place to express yourself authentically. If you pursue an intentional living, minimalist principles, and various decluttering and beautifying techniques, your home will not only find a balance between utility and presentation, but you will be giving yourself the chance to find happiness in your home.

Making My Space Work For Me

Creating a stress-free zone at home will be one fundamental way to find happiness and rest these days. Depending on your situation and resources, reevaluating and revamping your home space may require more time, energy, and funds, but not necessarily. Something as simple as organizing or decluttering may be all that you need to make your home feel comfy and secure. Of course, some will love the opportunity to redecorate, but small changes around your home will be just as welcome. The key is to find ways to make your living space your own.

Intentional Living and Minimalist Philosophy

Whenever I look at pictures of minimalist houses, I wonder how the owners survive with so few pieces of furniture and the all-white and beige tones. Is this kind of catalog-esque, stark space really for me? Over time, however, I began to realize that my understanding of minimalism was a little bit skewed by media representation of the lifestyle. I have since learned that minimalism is actually about maximizing your time and energy for intentional living.

Intentional living? How is that different from what I'm doing right now? The truth is that you might be like me, having a few ideas and dreams that I'm pursuing, but nothing much beyond that. Intentional living is all about clarifying what you want from life and going after those goals. In order to achieve personal development and meaningful experiences, you want to use your time and energy wisely. Why waste time cleaning and maintaining your possessions when you could be experiencing life?

Some people enjoy their books, knick-knacks, and creative pieces. But if you're not careful, your possessions will become a way for you to evaluate your status in the materialist game of ownership. The stress of keeping up with the Joneses next door eventually eats away at your sense of selfhood and happiness. Releasing yourself from the comparison game, therefore, is a great way to pursue personal expression.

As a result, minimalism doesn't always include large amounts of decluttering, although that can happen. It is more focused on promoting order and harmony in your home and creating a space for freedom and self-expression. This is why there are many different kinds of approaches to minimalism:

- Classic Minimalism: Less is more.

- Green Minimalism: Minimize your carbon footprint.

- Nomadic Minimalism: Free yourself for experiences.

- Spiritual Minimalism: Make a sanctuary.

It's time to reevaluate your life and assess your private spaces. What can you do to maximize your happiness and minimize negativity and fatigue? Let's have a look at a few home care tips.

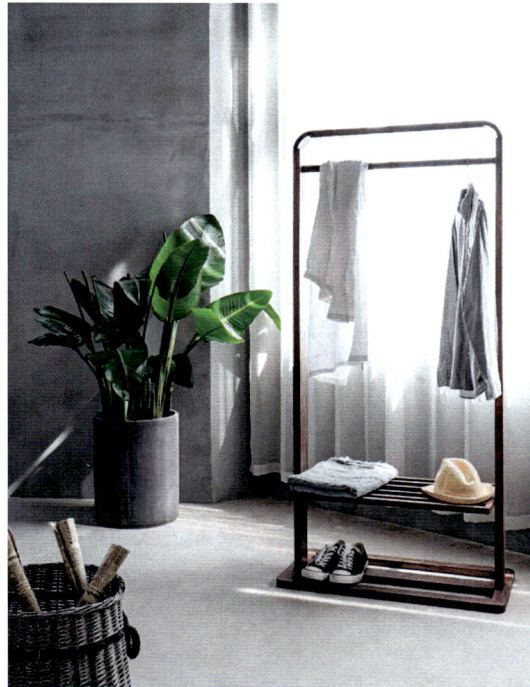

Decluttering Methods

You might be ready to start throwing stuff out. But before you start tossing stuff in garbage bags, you might want to consider strategizing how you go about decluttering. Following a decluttering method doesn't just give you focus or keep you motivated; it makes sure that you don't regret throwing something out later, causing you to go shopping again. Furthermore, many decluttering methods can be quite extreme (KonMari Method and Party Packing Method), so you may need to alter the steps for their decluttering methods or fuse ideas with other more achievable decluttering techniques.

The KonMari method. Marie Kondo, a Japanese cleaning consultant, has been in the business for a while but recently burst into popularity due to her Netflix show *Tidying Up with Marie Kondo*. Her famous question, "Does it spark joy?" is the lynchpin for her decluttering method. Heavily influenced by Japanese spirituality and culture, Kondo believes that your respect for your home and possessions will define what you own and what you let go of.

How to do the KonMari method:

1. Get ready to declutter all in one go! You should begin with a self-affirmative commitment before starting the process.

2. Keeping your ideal home in mind, use the KonMari list to understand what you need versus what you can let go of.

3. Declutter by category, not by room, following the KonMari list order exactly.

4. As you consider each item, be honest with yourself about whether you need it or whether it "sparks joy". If it isn't adding toward your ideal home, let it go.

5. Once you finish discarding, you should say a word of thanks for the items that have served you well before letting them go.

6. After getting the decluttered items out of your home, reorganize your living space.

The KonMari list:

1. Clothing: Go through each clothing item by sub-category (tops, bottoms, socks, shoes, etc) for each person in the house.

2. Books: Keep only the books that you absolutely need. Don't forget to go through your recipe or hobby book as well!

3. Papers: Throw out old or unnecessary receipts, bills, homework, projects, etc.

4. Miscellaneous: This is the largest category to tackle. You will have to go through various rooms of your house, cleaning out knick-knacks and odds and ends as well as other possessions.

5. Sentimental Items: Sort through personal writing or art projects as well as photographs, souvenirs, or heirlooms.

The Party Packing method. Ryan Nicodemus reached a state of crisis in his life that resulted in him going to his good friend Joshua Fields Millburn for help. Joshua, who was a practicing minimalist, suggested that Ryan restart his life from the ground up. The Party Packing Method was invented by Ryan and Joshua as a way for Ryan to dramatically rethink his life goals and possessions. Although it requires you to declutter all in one go as well as live out of boxes for up to a month, this dramatic change might be what you need to transform your perspective!

How to do the Party Packing method:

1. [optional] Throw a party with friends.

2. Together, pack everything you own up into boxes, bins, and packing wrap.

3. Don't leave out anything! Wrap even the furniture up!

4. Over the following weeks, only take out what you need to use, for practical, emotional, or other reasons.

5. After a month has passed, donate, sell, gift, or throw out anything left over still packed.

The Four Box method. Recommended by the famous minimalist Joshua Becker, this old-time tradition of decluttering still can be useful today. Less dramatic than the KonMari Method or the Party Packing Method, this decluttering technique allows you to take your time assessing what you need. This more flexible approach to decluttering is recommended for larger households.

How to do the Four Box Method:

1. Find four boxes that you can use for decluttering. They need to be the right size so that you can move them around or carry them easily.

2. Label each box one of the following: Storage, Toss, Donate/Sell, Keep.

3. Choose a room or a corner of a room and begin sorting items.

4. As you pick up an item, ask yourself some of the following questions:

    a. How often do I use this?

    b. Would I miss it if I threw it out?

    c. Should it be here?

5. When your boxes are full empty them right away!

    a. Trash: Put the items into a garbage bag right away and put them outside.

    b. Sell/Donate: Put the items into boxes and store them in the garage or the back of your car. Items you plan to sell should be photographed and advertised immediately.

    c. Storage: Place the items in this box into storage.

    d. Keep: Put the items away in the place where they belong.

The Day-by-Day Detox method. Jennifer Lifford shared her decluttering method, the 30-Day Clutter Detox Plan, on the Oprah Winfrey Show. Her technique can be modified to follow a 30-day challenge. All you have to do is focus on one area or one thing to declutter, such as your purse or your closet. Within a month, you will discover that your home is looking a bit more tidy and organized. This challenge is more doable for large homes and bigger families!

How to do the Day-by-Day Detox Method:

Day 1: Paperwork

Day 2: Front Entryway/Coat Closet

Day 3: Purse

Day 4: Cleaning Supplies

Day 5: Fridge and Freezer

Day 6: Pantry/Dry Food Storage

Day 7: Free-for-all

Day 8: Kitchen Cabinets

Day 9: Medicine Cabinet/First Aid Supplies

Day 10: Dining Area

Day 11: Entertainment Area

Day 12: Magazines and Books

Day 13: Junk Drawer

Day 14: Free-for-all

Day 15: Desk

Day 16: Bathroom Cabinets

Day 17: Linen Closet

Day 18: Makeup

Day 19: Jewelry

Day 20: Bedroom Closet

Day 21: Free-for-all

Day 22: Sock and Underwear Drawer

Day 23: Nightstand

Day 24: Kids' Toys

Day 25: Kids' Closets

Day 26: Craft Space

Day 27: Laundry Room

Day 28: Free-for-all

Day 29: Basement

Day 30: Garage

Day 31: Car

Make this list your own by switching things up or replacing different areas with spaces unique to your home!

The Swedish Death Cleaning method. From Sweden comes a very different yet just as mindful way of looking at your life and possessions. Like the Four Box Method, this can be achieved at your own pace. Döstädning, "death cleaning", is what Swedish people call decluttering after a person who has died. One way to lessen the impact of your stuff on other people's lives after you are gone is to declutter mindfully. Margareta Magnusson, in her book *The Gentle Art of Swedish Death Cleaning*, explains how this form of decluttering is about passing on a positive legacy, leaving behind only things that will hold meaning for your loved ones. Although this decluttering method is aimed at seniors, it is a good wake-up call for anyone.

How To Swedish Death Clean:

1. Think about what you want to achieve in life and what will make you happy.

2. Go through storage areas first, getting rid of obvious garbage.

3. Set aside items that may have value for friends and family.

4. Work through the rest of your home, starting with more hidden areas, like your closet.

5. Ask yourself these questions if you aren't sure whether to hold onto or let go of an item:

    a. What do I need to live happily?

    b. What do I want to pass on as my heritage?

    c. What things do I own that might be upsetting, embarrassing, or hurtful?

    d. What is important to me alone?

6. Leave sentimental items to the end (like journals, letters, and photographs). Place these in a chest or box where they can be stored safely.

7. The rest of the stuff that you don't want or need, you can gift, donate, or sell.

8. Talk with a friend or family member about how to dispose of the sentimental items after you die.

Keeping Cleaning Simple

When I get home from work, it can be hard to face the disorder that has accumulated over the past few days. I feel so tired, physically and mentally, I more often than not end up just procrastinating on my chores. By the time the weekend rolls around, things have gotten out of hand. As time went by, I began to realize that my habit of putting things off was making things worse. I decided to set up a small cleaning schedule for myself, one that would help me keep the craziness at bay.

It worked! You can try something like this out as well. Change it up, depending on the size of your home, whether you have a helpful family or not.

My cleaning schedule:

Daily

- Dishes
- Bed
- Kitchen counter and table
- Sinks
- Floors (sweeping)
- Bathroom surfaces and walls

Weekly

- Laundry
- Mirrors
- Floors (sweeping, vacuuming, and mopping)
- Appliances (wiping microwave/stove/coffee maker)
- Declutter (pantry, fridge, and other rooms)

Monthly

- Baseboards
- Vents
- Light fixtures
- Clean dishwasher, vacuum, laundry machines
- Curtains/blinds

Bi-Annually

- Large appliances (oven/fridge/freezer)
- Under/behind furniture
- Mattress
- Drains
- Garbage cans

Annually

- Chimney/fireplace
- Windows
- Gutters
- Carpets/upholstery

Simplifying the Art of Decor

If your home is decluttered, organized, and clean, it will be easier to see how you can express your taste and individuality through art and decor. Not all of us can afford major home renovations. That's why small changes can be a great start for your journey to a better home and a better you!

So, what kind of personal touches should you aim for? Here are some ways to revitalize your living spaces.

Make a statement with art. Finding the right art to hang on the wall can be difficult. An important thing to keep in mind is choosing art that shows emotions you want to feel or represents an aspect of yourself, whether it is an interest or part of your cultural heritage.

- Hang or place art, crafts, or other creative products you (or your children) have made around the house.
- Think about the size and textures of the art you place so that the room doesn't get too crowded.
- Support local artists by buying their art at local community sales.
- Try to find art or sculptures that express your cultural heritage.
- Showcase family photographs in collages or a wall of photographs.

Create a mood with lighting. Sometimes a room changes just by replacing the lightbulb with a different color or type of lighting. Warm lighting is less abrasive to your eyes. Think about the different ways you can add pop lighting to a room!

- Choose LED-type lights with warmer tones between 1000-3000k.

- Light candles or your (electric) fireplace for more organic warm lighting.

- Try out pop lightings, such as string lights, wax burners, or night lights.

- Invest in smart lighting, which allows you to change the colors of your lighting up depending on the occasion.

- Use task lighting, like desk/reading lamps, to set apart specific areas in your home

Feed the eye and the touch. When choosing art or fabrics, try to find a harmonious mix of color and texture. This will not only give your home a unique feel but also evoke a feeling of coziness and relaxation. If your furniture has simple solid colors, you can spice things up with the art and fabrics you place in the room! If your furniture set is already a statement piece, provide solid pop colors with the pillows and throws.

- Mix and match furniture so that your home feels more individual and 'you' than a catalog book.

- When choosing materials for home decor, mix it up with a combo of leather, ceramic, and wood.

- Consider using wooden antique furniture for an older, homey feel.

- Switch fabric styles between seasons. In the winter, use velvet or heavy draping for curtains. In the summer, opt for sheer linen.

- Decorate your walls and bedspreads with textured, woven, or quilted throws, blankets, and pillows.

Cultivate a hospitable home. It can be hard to make your home your own, especially if you have space limitations or a busy family life. You can start by analyzing what experience you want to create for guests when they visit. What emotions do you want them to have when they visit? This can help you define the hospitable experience you are invested in giving.

- Make little areas in your house where people can gather in nooks to chat privately.

- Have background soft jazz, classical, or ambient music going.

- Refresh the scents of your home. Try crowd-pleasers like cookie dough, flowers, or coffee beans.

- Provide slippers at the door.

- In the living room, group the seating closer to encourage the feeling of intimacy.

Bring the Outdoors Indoors. Checking in with the rhythms of earth through contact with nature boosts positive physical and mental health. As we get in touch with positive sensory experiences in nature, we can feel more grounded and prepared for the day ahead.

- Before choosing or placing plants, take notice of what sunlight you have in your home. Depending on what plants you choose, you will have to increase or limit sunlight exposure.

- Put larger plants in the corners of your rooms.

- If you have a balcony, porch, deck, or large windows, place plants that love sunlight around or on them.

- Allergic? Try getting faux greenery or dried flowers instead!

- Consider allergy-friendly plants: Kentia Palm, Aloe Vera, Bamboo Palm, Arginata, Dracaena, Philodendron

Many of these tips and tricks won't take a lot of time or energy. You might have to rethink how you are using your space and moving a few things around. On the other hand, maybe some of you are like me. I ended up having to seriously revamp my living space, rethinking what I needed and what was dragging me down. Once I figured out how to reorient my belongings and home, I felt free to spend my time the way I wanted in a place that was optimized to support and inspire me.

Seeking Sanctuary

What makes a home homey? What creates the feeling of coziness and safety for you? What relaxes and inspires you? What is going to give you energy? All of these questions need to be answered to maximize what your home can give you. I believe that you should consider the importance of an organized, intentional, clean, and beautiful space, and also completely rethink how you separate the areas of your home.

One of the problems I faced, for example, was my futon couch. I began to realize that I was spending too much of my free time lying on top of it instead of working on my projects, getting housework done, or even focusing on a good book. There was a very real connection in my head between my futon and Netflix. Moving my futon to the spare room in my apartment and getting a second-hand wingback chair was all the change-up that I needed to reorient my focus and energy. This doesn't mean that I stopped enjoying Netflix, but it gave me more room for my creative desk space and also helped me set aside my armchair area for reading and Netflix.

If you are like me and are finding yourself more trapped at home, setting different areas of your house aside for specific activities can help you form healthier boundaries. For example, consider where your "at home office" is. Is your desk in a corner of your bedroom or living room? You might want to think about ways to move it to a more separate area, such as another room. Setting up room divider alternatives or a kind of closeable desk that can signal the end of work might help you separate your work and home life even when you are working at home.

Similarly, I discovered that setting your bedroom aside for sleeping and relaxing helps you create boundaries physically and mentally. When I enter my room, I feel at peace. I am encouraged to unplug, so I am not distracted by work or social media notifications. There is space set aside in one corner for exercise, which I can easily access every morning. All of these decisions were designed to help me make better choices and have already improved my outlook on life. I encourage you to re-envision what home looks like for you and empower yourself with the energy and inspiration of a comfy sanctuary.

Chapter 5:

My Selfhood

After watching the 50th episode of my favorite TV show, I knew that something had to change. Although I had a lot of fun, the amount of time deciding what to watch was beginning to increase. More and more shows and stories became boring, and several hours of chilling with Netflix became less and less satisfying. Suddenly, waiting for the next season of my favorite shows began to feel like forever. What was I going to watch next?

Then, there was my phone. It was easy for me to uninstall Facebook, but I had a few games that I enjoyed when I wasn't busy with work or watching Netflix. Sometimes, I would focus on the game and just let the TV run in the background as comforting white noise. However, I began to realize that the small budget I had set for myself in terms of spending on games began to feel tighter than usual. The games were becoming grindy, forcing the invested player base to spend more money. Rampant monetization began to make it impossible for me to enjoy the simple pleasures of a decorating or tap-tap adventure game.

How was I going to spend my time? If I can't enjoy reruns anymore if social media is too toxic if my favorite mobile games are overly monetized, what should I focus on instead? It took me a while to figure out the answer. It came to me one day while I was spending some time scheduling. As I thought through a problem, I idly started to doodle in the corner of my page. The mindless exercise somehow calmed me down and before I knew it, half the page was filled in with squiggles. I realized that the simple act of doodling helped me focus in a good way and kept me feeling serene as I figured out a solution.

The moment spent doodling reminded me of the times I had spent drawing at night in my sketchbooks and journals. Art has always been a way for me to work through my emotions. On some level, just concentrating on the drawing took me away from the situations and thoughts that were bothering me. For a moment, I was able to focus on one thing and celebrate the end product afterward. In the process, I found serenity and the ability to look at the situation with new eyes.

That's when I knew that the answer to my problem lay in my ability to express myself. Although gaming and watching TV is fun, another great way to spend my time would be to use my type of creativity to explore my emotions, achieve small improvements, and share my art in my home. There are many ways to cultivate creative expression. I knew that perhaps returning to art would be the answer. It was!

In the same way, you can achieve personal growth and positivity through expanding your creative energies. As you finish each small project, you will find yourself growing with confidence and motivation. There will be opportunities to rediscover parts of yourself emotionally and mentally as well! In those moments of hard work, you may be able to set aside other life situations and relax in a more productive, active kind of way that will also inspire and motivate you. I highly recommend, therefore, that you consider the ways that you can transform your mindset and interests so that you can explore the internal and external worlds of your personhood and experiences.

Taking Stock

The first part of any journey to self-actualization begins with an exploration of the self, where you begin to confront with honesty who you truly are. It isn't always easy because there are going to be parts of yourself that we don't like. There are going to be moments where you might feel discouraged. However, right around the corner are opportunities for you to discover both about yourself and about the possibilities that life can bring you!

When it comes to thinking about who you are, there are many ways to go about it. One of the best strategies is to consider your advantages and flaws. What might your strengths and weaknesses be? What are you good at doing? What do you struggle with? For some people, listing strengths is easy; for others, all they see are the flaws. It is crucial to maintain a positive attitude as you consider the resources that you have been given, whether it is a character trait or a natural skill.

The Basic Approach

The easiest way to start thinking about yourself is to set aside a page in your journal. I started with this exercise because it helped me brainstorm ideas about myself. Drawing a line down the center, I named one column "Strengths" and the other column "Weaknesses". Over the next few days, I watched myself and spoke with close friends who could give me some perspective as well.

I focused quite a bit on the personality traits or skills that I was good at. For weaknesses, I kept the list to less than 10 items. I felt like it was important that I didn't feel too overwhelmed by what I had to work on. These two lists provided a good foundation for getting an idea of what inner resources and skills I could draw on in the future.

You can consider this list of character strengths as a good starting point for you to consider.

- Love
- Kindness
- Perseverance
- Gratitude

- Optimism
- Humour
- Purpose
- Self-control
- Humility
- Forgiveness
- Fair
- Leadership
- Teamwork
- Perspective
- Curiosity
- Creativity
- Bravery

However, strengths aren't just about the person you are but also what you can do. Therefore, you can consider writing down phrases like "Good at. . ." or "Able to. . ." `` Try to be as creative as you can when you list all of the things you feel confident doing.

On the other hand, when taking stock of your weaknesses, you can consider some of the opposites of these strengths. For example, if you struggle with not being creative, you can write down "lack of creativity". If you decide to focus on one or two things you think you could work on, do just that! Overwhelming yourself with the negative is a sure-fire way to slow you down and demotivate you!

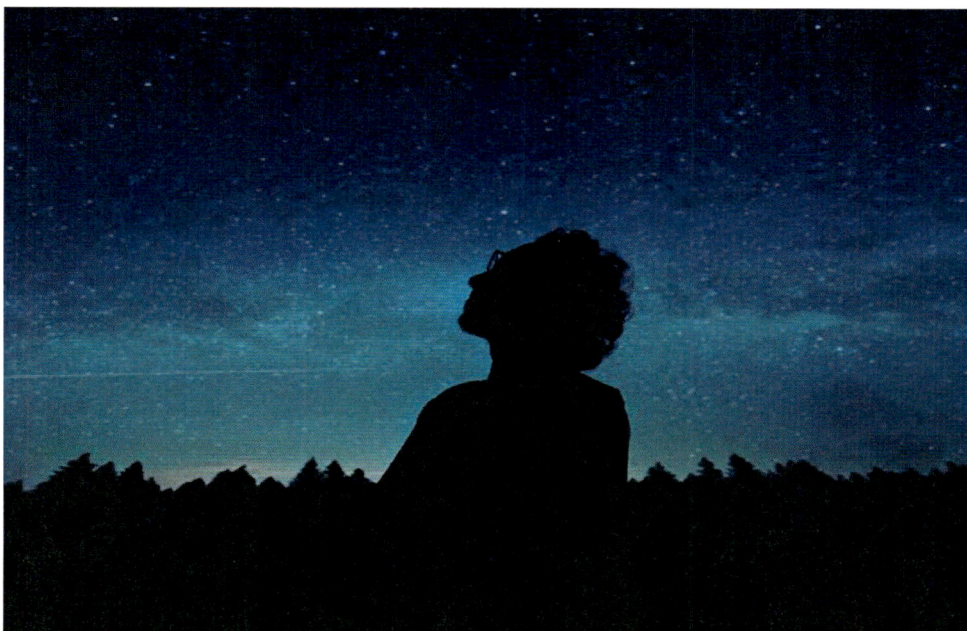

Once you have a list of what you feel comfortable and uncomfortable doing, you will have a better perspective of yourself, which you can then apply to your plans and strategies during meditation and journaling times. For example, I realized that I'm not that great at math, so moving forward, I decided to get help with budgeting through a software solution on my phone. This way, I could keep track of expenses even though I struggle with handling numbers well. However, I realized that I am a very creative person, so I decided to use my creativity as a way to express myself in my spare time as well as come up with alternative solutions to problems I hadn't yet solved. In a similar way, you might realize there are ways to use your strengths to your advantage as you work toward positive life choices and personal development.

SWOT Analysis

Another common way of self-analysis, often used in business or career development, is the SWOT Analysis system. SWOT is an acronym that stands for:

- Strengths: character traits, abilities, and skills that you have

- Weaknesses: areas where you may be less skilled or have less positive traits

- Opportunities: possibilities or strategies that you can use to achieve your goals or personal growth

- Threats: things that will stop you from achieving your goals or personal growth

Given how goal-oriented this self-analysis system is, the SWOT process begins with choosing a goal you want to focus on. I had a goal to balance a healthy budget over the year. Once I set that goal for myself, I analyzed my strengths and weaknesses, as well as the opportunities and threats that might factor in this process.

Strength: Creativity and curiosity. I knew that these two character traits would help me figure out what I needed to do to balance my budget for the year. I also felt that I was tech-savvy, so that I could look at alternative software to help me plan for financial success.

Weakness: Not so great at math. Since I realized that math wasn't my strong suit, I knew that deep-diving into spreadsheets and formulas wasn't an option.

Opportunities: My phone. I knew that I could find an app in the store that would help me figure out how to keep an eye on expenditure. Sure enough, after researching a bit online and reading through reviews, I decided on the one that would work for me!

Threats: Stress and poor habits. One of the things I pinpointed as a problem was stress. This is because when I'm stressed, my go-to is ordering some fast food or snacks. Under stress, I'm less likely to spend time cooking healthy meals. So I began to plan ways to mitigate this problem by revisiting the way I prepared meals. I also knew that remembering to input information into my phone would take time. As a result, I worked toward forming better habits when it came to cataloging expenditures and checking in on my bank balance.

Although SWOT Analysis is often used in terms of business orientation and career, you can keep these four points in mind when you assess yourself in light of the goals that you have chosen for yourself. Knowing what you want and need is not enough. You have to be ready to empower yourself to get there! With the help of these tools, you will be poised for success!

Reorienting Your Mindset

I have a coworker friend who constantly beats himself up. His eye for detail and his love of precision is a double-edged sword. Since he is so meticulous, he often struggles with a perfectionist streak. When things are less than perfect, he struggles with keeping perspective and seeing the positive side of a situation. After most of our coworkers had left the Zoom meeting, we hung out for a bit to catch up on a project we were working on.

Halfway through, my friend admitted, "It's tough, you know? I always feel like it's never enough. There's always something I have to tweak or finish. I know that if we were at work, you would be tearing it out of my hands. . . I guess I need that more than I thought."

His admission made me realize that I wasn't the only one struggling with getting used to working at home. Other people at work were also having a tough time. In the case of some, they were unable to accept their limitations. They needed the input and the boundaries set by other people in their life. This realization challenged me a little and got me thinking about how we view ourselves and the world. It isn't always easy to forgive yourself or treat yourself well, but there is a balance that we should pursue between love and truth in our lives.

The Impact of Love

Self-compassion and self-respect are rooted in one basic idea: you are valuable. As you view your life, consider the idea that you have value, not only as a human being but also for your unique blend of strengths and flaws. Your experiences and personality have formed a unique perspective. You need to stand firm in the understanding that you as an individual matter. As this belief becomes real for you, you will learn how to be kinder to yourself as well as encourage yourself to make positive choices for change.

Learn to forgive yourself. Messing up is difficult. Not only might a difficult situation be made even harder due to a mistake or due to lack of skill, but your emotional and mental energies can take a hit when you dwell on failure. This is why it is important to understand the importance of forgiveness, not only for others but also for yourself. When you forgive yourself, you are moving from negative emotions into a more positive mindset, which will help you solve the problem and avoid the same mistake in the future.

Recognize that you deserve better. Understanding that you have value leads to a sense of dignity and self-respect that can help you say no to bad habits or poor choices. Many times our go-to during times of stress is unhealthy, so it's a good idea to listen to the internal voice inside you that might be encouraging you in other, more helpful directions. The quiet voice within might be saying something like "Is this actually helpful?" or "Will this change anything?" If you are feeling hesitant, perhaps you need to look for other options beyond the chips or cigarettes, or remote control that you are reaching for.

The Power of Truth

Hand in hand with love, truth plays another role in our lives. When honesty is coupled with courage, we begin to gain perspective. We can see ourselves and our life for what it truly is. If we can recognize our limitations and our abilities, we will be better equipped to strategize for the creation of happiness and fulfillment in life. How can we empower ourselves with perspective? Let's have a look at the forgotten truths of Stoicism!

Stoicism is an ancient Greek philosophy that has gotten a bad rap. I was a bit confused about the concepts of Stoicism because all I could remember about it was something about not showing emotion. I was way off! This ancient philosophy is a powerful way of viewing yourself, encouraging positive characteristics like wisdom, self-control, justice, and courage. In a nutshell, stoicism encourages you to recognize what you can change and what you can't. By focusing on what you can change, this belief empowers you to transform yourself and the areas in your life that you can change, while using your strengths to weather any difficult storm that is ongoing in your life.

As mentioned before, taking a moment to analyze yourself and your situation might feel counterintuitive at first, but, as you gain perspective on the challenge or issues before you, you will feel empowered to overcome the odds. Unbalanced stoicism can result in harsh standards that you require of yourself and other people. However, positive stoicism provides wisdom and discipline on the path to happiness and fulfillment. Consider these questions as your journal and meditate to help achieve balance and perspective.

- What can I do to make this situation better?
- If I can't change what is going on, how can I minimize the negative impact?
- What is the worst-case scenario? What is the best-case scenario?
- What practical steps will move me toward a positive future?
- What is important *right now*?

Exploring the World

Though I knew it was important to reorient my mindset about who I am—learning to love and respect *me*, I felt like gaining perspective on myself was difficult. I began to look for ways to express myself and explore my emotions and thoughts, which led me to revisit art. I became more certain than ever that learning something new or working on a hobby was a healthy way to use my energy. I discovered quite a few reasons why investing time in a hobby, skill, or interest is crucial.

Relieve Stress and Decrease Depression. Running away from issues in your life rarely solves anything. However, limited time spent with books, video games, and puzzles provides a way for us to gain confidence and exercise our brains. Other hobbies can also temporarily shift our focus into creative self-expression that allows us to process our emotions and regain serenity. As a result, many forms of hobbies, when approached with balance, can help you cope with stress.

Replace Negative Activities. Although enjoying a night on the sofa with Netflix or a video game isn't always bad, sometimes we can get too caught up in our phones or TV watching other people's lives instead of investing in our own. Other unhelpful activities look differently for each of us, whether it is time spent pacing, overeating, or even over-socializing.

Improve Memory and Concentration. When we learn new skills, such as a hobby or another language, the pathways of neurons in our brains are renewed. This discourages cognitive decline, increasing our ability to remember and concentrate in other areas of our lives.

Create Confidence and Accomplishment. After learning something new, experiencing creative energy, or finishing a project, you may feel a burst of energy, inspiration, and confidence. When you share your experiences or the finished project with your friends, you will naturally feel happy and excited. If you receive positive feedback from your family, friends, or interest group, you will feel more ready to take on other projects and tasks. These feelings will naturally impact how you view other situations in life. Therefore, the pride and joy of completing a project can never be underestimated. After finishing your art piece, woodwork, or musical composition, be sure to share it with family and friends or others online. The unique identity that is representative of yourself is sure to be an encouragement or thoughtful challenge to the world at large!

Express Yourself. When we explore our emotions and ideas in art or craftwork, we are engaging with a unique way to express ourselves. Even if you are working through a tutorial, the skills that you pick up will one day be used to reveal your individuality. Even with the internet, we may feel unable to express ourselves. Either we haven't found a good community to connect with or we may feel like our point of view isn't accepted. Through creative expression, you will be able to express yourself and share it through gifts or home decor touches.

Receive Additional Income. Once you feel confident enough about your abilities, you can always explore options to monetize your hobby as a side option for income. These days, opening a digital storefront offers an opportunity for those with a budding interest in entrepreneurship.

Transition Easier into Retirement. When I look forward to my life as a retiree, I wonder how I'm going to use my spare time. It reminds me of my mother's struggles with empty nest syndrome. For a while, she had a hard time figuring out what she was interested in and what she wanted to invest her time and energy into. Starting a hobby earlier in your life provides you with a readymade activity to sink into as a retiree, relieving the stress of transition into retirement.

Create boundaries. Working at home might be hard for you because you can't focus with noisy kids, cuddly pets, or distracting partners. On the other hand, you might be struggling to draw the line after a full workday. Without structured scheduling, you might find it hard to turn your computer off at night, stop answering emails, or take a break to sit down and enjoy dinner. Setting yourself up with a hobby encourages structure in your life. Knowing that you have to get to the gym or hang out with your reading club promotes healthy boundaries, limiting your involvement with work within reasonable hours.

Foster social connections. As lockdowns end and quarantine restrictions are eased, you might be more than ready to hang out with your friends. What are you going to do? Spend more time indoors? Or are you ready to try something new? Instead of settling for Netflix and chill, try out a new hobby with your friend! If you are discovering that meaningful connections are missing from your life, a good idea might be to get plugged into an interest group. With a shared focus on creative expression, you will not only be encouraged but also inspired!

Find inspiration. Many times when we face a challenging situation, we might be unsure of how to go about solving the problem. Perhaps our first few attempts are unsuccessful. Where are we going wrong? Well, one of the issues might be that our approaches are too focused on what we learned in the past. Over-reliance on past experiences can limit our ability to problem-solve. However, through creative expression, we are often tested in terms of innovation, flexibility, and creativity. The processes of learning a new skill or improving in a hobby can lead to an increase in inspiration. We will be more open to thinking outside the box in other areas of our life!

Considering all of these reasons why you should start investing some time and energy into a hobby or interest, you might be wondering, "Where do I start?" Good question. I began to look back into my past and considered what worked for me before. However, there are a few other ways to explore the world around you.

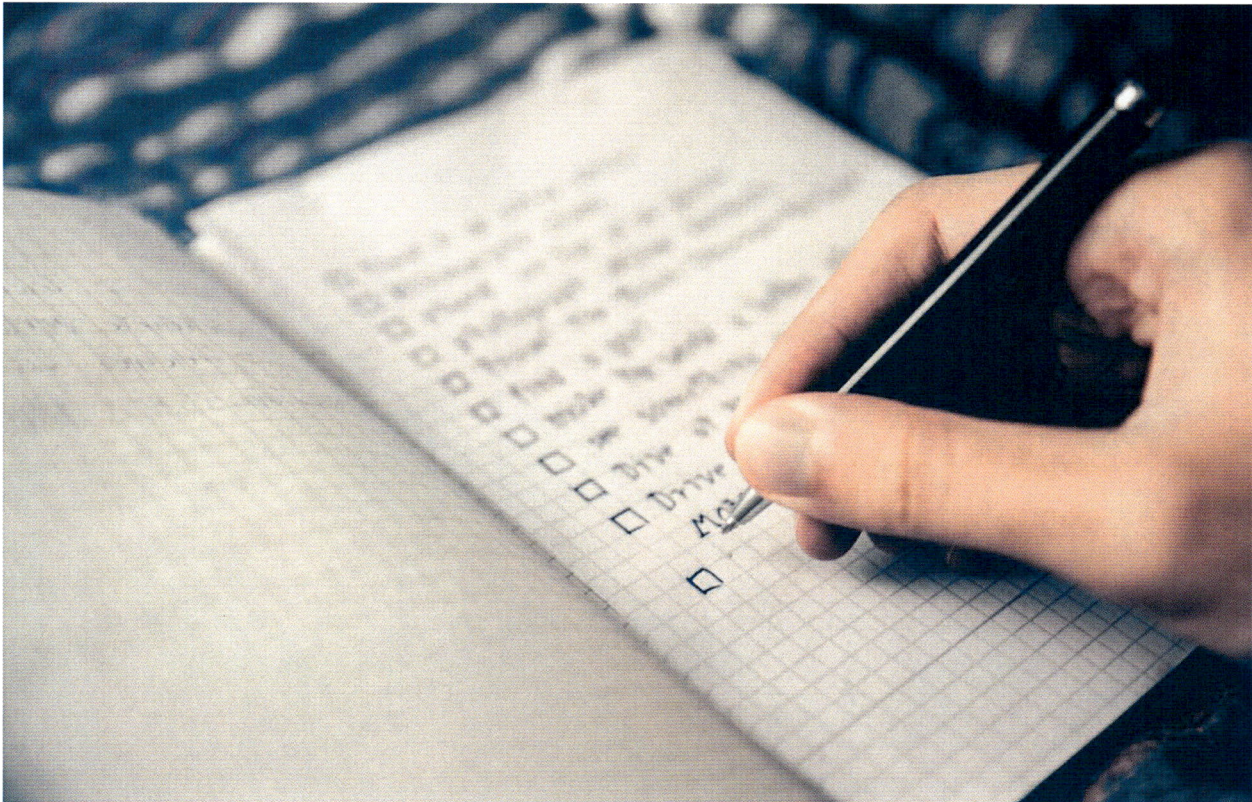

Create a bucket list. Bucket lists set goals you want to reach before "you kick the bucket". The amazing thing about bucket lists is that they can open up possibilities as you consider the many different activities you can participate in. Ranging from very physical experiences to more cerebral ones, comprehensive bucket lists can be a great springboard for ideas. It is important to make your bucket list personal, but reading bucket list ideas is a good way to get inspired! Check out these examples!

- Go on an adventure
  - Surfing
  - Ride a zipline
  - Hang gliding
  - Skydiving
  - Snowboarding/skiing
  - Snorkeling
  - Whitewater rafting
- Get in touch with nature
  - Go to a rodeo
  - Climb a volcano

- o Feed wild animals
- o Work at a pet shelter
- o Go horseback riding
- o Swim with dolphins
- o Camping
- Connect with people
  - o Attend/hold a reunion
  - o Make a new friend
  - o Forgive someone
  - o Reconnect with an old friend
  - o Set up coffee dates with close friends
  - o Join a local art or hobby club
- Expand your entertainment tastes
  - o Take part in a masquerade
  - o Hold a murder mystery dinner
  - o Attend a gallery opening
  - o Go to a poetry reading
  - o Enjoy a concert or recital
  - o Visit a festival or fair (Renaissance or music)
  - o Host a karaoke evening
- Explore the world of cooking
  - o Go to a beer or soup festival
  - o Hold a tea party
  - o Host a bake-off or potluck
  - o Learn how to create food or latte art
  - o Make your own cocktail
  - o Try out new restaurants
  - o Go fruit picking at a farm

Surf the Net. One of the greatest resources you have is the internet. Unfortunately, if you are like me, you might be struggling with making the internet work for you. The risk of getting caught up in the noise and pressures of social media is high. It isn't just the constant debates, news bytes, or clickbait that causes additional stress, but also the unending stream of advertising that keeps tabs of what you are texting and talking about or what you are searching for on Google. You might feel like the time has come to opt-out of the internet entirely, but I think that might limit your ability to connect intentionally online with people who share interests with you. Also, if you know where to look, you can find great guides and tips for pretty much any hobby or skill that you are trying to improve!

Learning and studying skills online is one of the best ways to use the internet. With online tutorials and guides everywhere, whether on Pinterest, Instagram, or YouTube, you will find a lot of support as you learn new techniques and skills. When I was trying to figure out how to draw hands more realistically, I found some great tutorials on Udemy and SkillShare. Other sites, such as Master Class Online, might be more pricey, but they will connect you with the best and most talented in the field, whether you are learning how to compose music or write a book.

Another positive aspect of the internet is the opportunity to share your experiences and end product. Popular sites such as YouTube, Tumblr, or DeviantArt provide comprehensive ways to interface with fellow artists and hobbyists. If you are a writer, online novel sharing sites, such as Wattpad and Inkitt enable you to connect with an audience and get constructive feedback. If you find a supportive forum or online community like Discord or Livejournal, you will be able to not only enjoy the hobby of your choice but also build intentional relationships around shared experiences!

Lastly, when used correctly, the internet offers you an opportunity to open and walk through the door of exploration, discover new ideas, inspiration, and guides that can propel you further into the world of creativity. Sometimes you need a change. You need to try something new. For example, let's say a person is used to playing one kind of video game all the time. Perhaps if they watched a Twitch streamer introduce a new game, they would be open to trying out something new, something challenging. In this way, the internet can seem overwhelming. You might wonder, "Where do I start?" However, with sites like YouTube or Twitch, you can spend a few hours cruising top ten lists or watching hobbyists introduce their craft, opening your limited vista into broader horizons.

Explore options in your community. Some bucket lists can feel extreme, but connecting with a community center or local college might be another great option. Usually, you can find a welcoming, low-key interest groups, seminars, or instructional sessions through local recreation centers. You will be surprised at where you can find hobbyists!

I remember this one time I was talking with my mom. She told me about a day she went shopping later at night with my dad and younger sister. While at the mall, they passed by the board game store to see if there was something my younger sister would like. They discovered a board gaming club instead. Once a week, my mother told me, players of all ages gather to play various board games together. The atmosphere was super chill. My mother, who was never interested in board games, felt impressed by the dedication of the gaming session hosts.

This memory always stuck with me, reminding me that my people are out there. It was just a matter of me finding them. At this point, you might already have a few ideas percolating. You might be thinking that there is something that has been catching your eye or piquing your interest. If you still aren't sure, check out some of the different options below!

The arts. Listening to talented and skilled friends talking about making art can be a bit intimidating and overwhelming. It's important to keep in mind that your journey to intentional self-expression is just that—your journey. When you return to creating art or begin to explore artistic possibilities, don't let yourself be held back by expectations that might be coming from without or within. Being patient with yourself and learning through experience is part and parcel of learning a new art form, and these approaches you cultivate can be utilized in other areas of your life. This is why when it comes to exploring your artistic expression, don't let your options become restricted in how you use the art medium. As a hobbyist, you are allowed to go at your own pace and push boundaries!

- Photography
- Digital Art
- Sketching
- Painting
- Coloring
- Playing a musical instrument
- Musical composition
- Dancing
- Acting

Crafting. Not a lot of people think of crafting when they think about therapeutic art, but for a long time, craftwork has been an important medium for cultural and individual expression. Knitting, for example, has proven to help people cope with stress and ease symptoms of depression. The amazing thing about crafting is how it requires creativity but often produces practical items, whether it is a restored table or a cozy scarf. If you feel a bit daunted by the cost or skill required by "high art", try out a craft instead!

- Crocheting/Knitting
- Sewing
- Quilting
- Knot Tying
- Woodburning
- Candlemaking
- Carpentry
- Antique Restoration

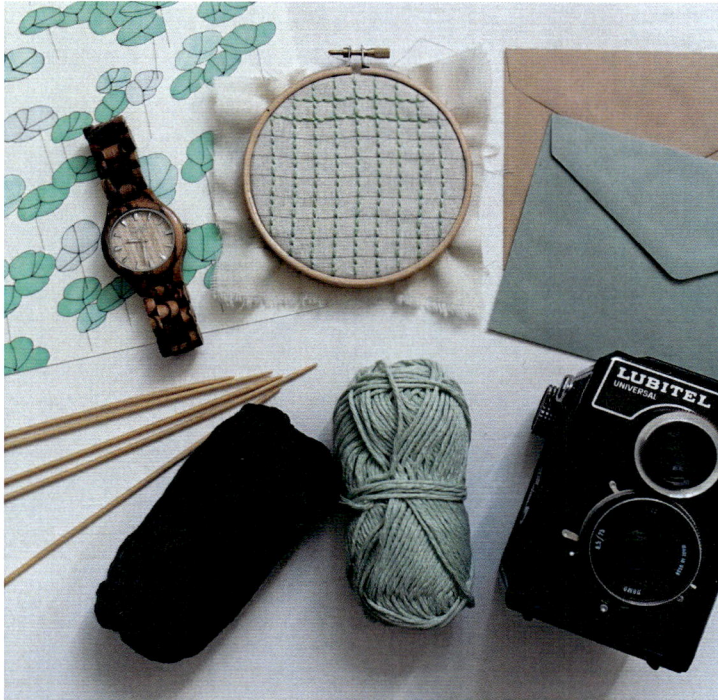

Physical activities. Not everyone is going to find energy or inspiration from arts and crafts. You might need to get outdoors or outside, where you can find energizing experiences that push you to your limits. Whether you enjoy volunteering or pursue fitness, physical activities are a great way to limit your work hours at home and get you moving, which is always great for your physical and mental health. These kinds of goals might push your physical limits, but they will provide positive memories of accomplishment that will carry forward into other areas of life.

- Volunteering at a school, library, or pet shelter
- Motorcycling
- Biking
- Exercising
- Fantasy Sports
- Sports
- Yoga
- Martial Arts
- Water sports
- Lifting Weights

So many ways to spend your time! It can be easy to limit therapeutic creativity to the arts, crafts, or sports, but modernity and technology provide many other popular ways to spend your time. Some of these hobbies might not produce an outcome you would link to personal growth, but many do still require a healthy level of concentration, problem-solving, and creativity to do well. Whether you are trying out a new recipe or learning how to use C#, the time spent achieving self-determined goals will be sure to result in less stress and more confidence in the future!

- Lego Building
- Puzzle-solving (crosswords, sudoku, logic puzzles)
- Cards
- Programming
- Reading
- Blogging
- Genealogy Hunting
- Cooking

Realizing Your Expressive Power

Accepting your creative agency is a crucial step to positive empowerment. As you explore your individual perspective and unique take on life, you are better able to confront emotions of all varieties and navigate problems in new ways. Your journey to authentic expression will provide you with self-respect and self-confidence. With inspiration and creativity made routine in your life, you will feel more ready to take on challenges that lie before you.

After many years of focusing on my schooling and career, returning to the simple hobby of drawing seemed strange at first. Buying cheap pencils at my local art store and a simple sketchbook didn't feel like a momentous occasion. Spending time listening to music for inspiration and drawing small sketches was, I thought, just another way to fill out my schedule. A few weeks later, when I showed some of my drawings to my friend, I realized how far I had come. My art wasn't perfect, but as I allowed myself to experiment and express how I was feeling, I began to realize that these experiences were important. My friend could feel what was coming across on the page. That's when I realized that pursuing creative expression didn't have to just belong to professionals. All of us, I realized, have the capacity to create. We can all discover new opportunities to rethink possibilities, to think outside the box, to overcome challenges, to be ourselves.

Can crocheting doilies or solving a crossword help? Will I rediscover truths about myself volunteering in a pet shelter or climbing a mountain? It sounds kind of crazy, I know, but these seemingly insignificant changes can transform your life. If you pursue self-analysis and self-expression, you will be able to understand what makes you happy and chase after it. Through the pursuit of a hobby, you can learn how to recognize your strengths and weaknesses. This offers you an opportunity to maximize your time and energy so that you will be able to strategize on how to reach your goals and achieve happiness and fulfillment in the process.

Conclusion

I know the walls of my home very well. So do you! After looking out of the same few windows over and over at the same scenery, it's hard not to feel trapped. Trying to escape by gaming on your phone, watching Netflix, or surfing social media only gets you so far, unfortunately.

At first, being able to see what your friends are up to is encouraging and exciting, but over time, as the debates over the pandemic, politics, and other hot topics begin to heat up, negativity and toxicity begin to derail your emotions and focus. Instead of making meaningful connections online, you find yourself focused on debating or comparing yourself with unknown people online or barely familiar acquaintances. Perhaps at some point, you caught yourself wondering whether this is all worth it. . .?

With your energies divided or drained, the answer is probably 'no'. Your work-life begins to feel more difficult. Maintaining routine feels impossible. Your home seems to be spiraling out of control. And your mental and physical health begins to suffer as well.

I'm glad to say that this doesn't have to be the case. You have what it takes to transform yourself and your world. Relying on your strengths and skills, you can rediscover the ways to leverage your time, energy, and resources to find happiness even during the most difficult times!

Journey to the Ideal Self

To make the journey to your ideal self, you need to keep in mind five important concepts. If you develop these characteristics in your life, you will find the inner resources you need to achieve happiness and health moving forward.

Self-compassion. There is a lot of talk these days about the importance of loving yourself. However, self-compassion is more than just loving yourself; it includes going easy on yourself when times get tough. Be understanding. Be kind. Allow yourself time to bounce back when you let yourself down. Without self-compassion, you will end up treating yourself like a tyrant and becoming the person you were trying to avoid.

Self-respect. Loving yourself requires self-respect because if you do not believe you are loveable or valuable, you aren't going to treat yourself well. Self-respect is the necessary ingredient to positive choices because it provides a foundational belief that we deserve more. Tell yourself that you deserve better: a better home, a better job, a better you! Don't settle for less. Instead, work toward the best version of your life that you want to see.

Self-awareness. It can take some time to understand yourself. You are the one living your life, so you know the most about yourself - or do you? With this mindset, you are not only going to understand what fallback responses you prefer in every phase of life, but you will also understand the motivations behind your actions. In this way, self-awareness plays an important part in understanding what you need to do to change habits or resolve conflicts. Spend time alone and learn to face honestly the person in the mirror.

Self-determination. In times of conflict, rumors, and misinformation, it can be hard to feel motivated. You might not feel like you can change anything that is going on around you. However, if you cultivate self-determination, you are harnessing your inner strength and perseverance to weather all storms. Use positive self-affirmations to propel you, uplifting and motivating you as you move toward your dreams and life of happiness.

Self-actualization. The final product of your hard work is the achievement of your ideal self, called actualization. As you work toward this goal, times might get difficult, but knowing that your growth and health are being cared for will give you a sense of serenity and happiness you will not find easily elsewhere. Whatever else is going on in the world, you will feel empowered to transform the corner of the world you are in.

How am I going to achieve all this? Well, all of the previous chapters hold the practical strategies and mindsets I need to develop as I move forward. I have to take time to be alone and assess what I want from life. Knowing what I need and breaking my goals down into achievable steps is half of the battle. The rest involves pursuing intentional living, keeping focused on my daily needs, and building meaningful relationships. With each small achievement, I have learned to celebrate, cultivating gratitude and happiness instead of guilt, fear, and shame. I encourage you to get out of the comparison game as well. If that means you have to take social media breaks or curate your friend's list, by all means, do what you have to do. As you transform your environment, you will also discover the inner reserves you never knew before.

The Path to Happiness

Waking up is never easy, but today felt just a bit better than the day before. I still love to hit the snooze button a few times, but at least when I finally crawl out of bed, I know the routine. Halfway through my early morning yoga stretches, I start to come alive. After showering and completing my morning routine, I review the plans I had set in place the night before over a cup of coffee and a small pre-planned breakfast.

Yes! I nod to myself. *I know I can do this.* I'm already looking forward to getting my list done because I've already prepared a small reward for myself in the evening.

Outside, the heavy clouds are parting here and there. The gray is slowly giving way to warm rays of sunlight streaking down. Glancing at the weather forecast, it's calling for rain, so I grab an umbrella with my cardigan and prepare to go out.

Although it's the weekend, I have a whole day of errands planned. There's shopping to do. Some light cleaning. Some preparation for work on Monday. It's OK though. I know I've got this.

Making my way out to the sidewalk, I notice the droplets of water on the green bushes. The pavement is darkened and splotchy with drying rain. I glance upward. The rain has stopped. For now. The day may turn out to be perfect, or it might not. Either way, I knew that things would turn out fine. A horn lightly honks. I smile and run to it. My friend is there, already waiting for me. My day has only just begun!

References

Ackerman, C. E. (2018, August 6). *What is Self-Expression and How to Foster It? (20 Activities + Examples)*. PositivePsychology.com. https://positivepsychology.com/self-expression/

Adams, K. (2019). *Journal Writing: A Short Course – The Center for Journal Therapy*. Journaltherapy.com. https://journaltherapy.com/journal-cafe-3/journal-course/

Agarwal, Dr. P. (2018, July 30). 5 Ways To Overcome Online Social Media Fatigue For Mental Well-Being. *Forbes*. https://www.forbes.com/sites/pragyaagarwaleurope/2018/07/30/5-ways-to-overcome-online-social-media-fatigue-for-mental-well-being/?sh=5404aff1cfaf

Anello, C. (2020, April 3). *The Happiness Project One-Sentence Journal: A Five-Year Record by Gretchen Rubin*. The Strategist; The Strategist. https://nymag.com/strategist/article/best-gratitude-journals.html

AnjaHome. (2020, December 2). *Minimalist Bullet Journal: How To Create The One For 2021 - AnjaHome*. AnjaHome. https://anjahome.com/minimalist-bullet-journal/

Ankrom, S. (2021). *Deep Breathing Exercises to Reduce Anxiety*. Verywell Mind. https://www.verywellmind.com/abdominal-breathing-2584115

Aswell, S. (2019, January 8). *I Use This 5-Minute Therapy Technique Every Day for My Anxiety*. Healthline; Healthline Media. https://www.healthline.com/health/mental-health/self-talk-exercises

Babauta, L. (2014, August 11). *How to Find Your Life Purpose: An Unconventional Approach - zen habits*. Zen Habits. https://zenhabits.net/life-purpose/

Barcelo, C. (2019, November 29). *woman doing yoga*. Unsplash.com; Unsplash. https://unsplash.com/photos/nqUHQkuVj3c

Becker, J. (2009a, July 29). *More Time for the Things That Matter Most*. Becoming Minimalist. https://www.becomingminimalist.com/benefit-things-that-matter-most/

Becker, J. (2009b, July 29). *More Time for the Things That Matter Most*. Becoming Minimalist. https://www.becomingminimalist.com/benefit-things-that-matter-most/

Becker, J. (2011, June 20). *What Is Minimalism?* Becoming Minimalist. https://www.becomingminimalist.com/what-is-minimalism/#:~:text=MINIMALISM%20IS%20OWNING%20FEWER%20POSSESSIONS,those%20things%20that%20matter%20most

Becker, J. (2012a, November 9). *How to Declutter Your Home: 10 Creative Decluttering Tips*. Becoming Minimalist. https://www.becomingminimalist.com/creative-ways-to-declutter/

Becker, J. (2012b, December 28). *Benefits of Minimalism: 21 Benefits of Owning Less*. Becoming Minimalist. https://www.becomingminimalist.com/minimalism-benefits/

Becker, J. (2019, August 29). *What Makes a Home Beautiful*. Becoming Minimalist. https://www.becomingminimalist.com/beautiful-home/

Bertelli, G. (2016, June 22). *green and black yarns with round brown watch and black Lubitel camera*. Unsplash.com; Unsplash. https://unsplash.com/photos/E25HcrW2Xlc

BetterHelp. (2013). *Professional Counseling With A Licensed Therapist*. Betterhelp.com. https://www.betterhelp.com/

BH&G Editors. (2016, February 23). *A Whole-House Cleaning Schedule You'll Actually Stick To*. Better

Homes & Gardens; Better Homes & Gardens. https://www.bhg.com/homekeeping/house-cleaning/tips/whole-house-cleaning-schedule/

Bhandari, S. (2003, February 10). *How to Get Help for Mental Health*. WebMD; WebMD. https://www.webmd.com/anxiety-panic/mental-health-tests-you-take

Blanner, J. (2020, February). *How to Make Your Home Feel Warm and Cozy (Even if You're a Minimalist)*. Julie Blanner. https://julieblanner.com/cozy/

Bradt, S. (2010, November 11). *Wandering mind not a happy mind*. Harvard Gazette; Harvard Gazette. https://news.harvard.edu/gazette/story/2010/11/wandering-mind-not-a-happy-mind/

Bray, B. (2019, March 10). *Maslow's Hierarchy of Needs and Blackfoot (Siksika) Nation Beliefs | Rethinking Learning*. Barbarabray.net. https://barbarabray.net/2019/03/10/maslows-hierarchy-of-needs-and-blackfoot-nation-beliefs/

Brewer, J. (2019, December 5). *How to Break Up with Your Bad Habits*. Harvard Business Review. https://hbr.org/2019/12/how-to-break-up-with-your-bad-habits

Budget Dumpster. (2015a, June 24). *How to Declutter Your Home: A Ridiculously Thorough Guide*. Budgetdumpster.com; Budget Dumpster. https://www.budgetdumpster.com/resources/how-to-declutter-your-home.php

Budget Dumpster. (2015b, June 24). *How to Declutter Your Home: A Ridiculously Thorough Guide*. Budgetdumpster.com; Budget Dumpster. https://www.budgetdumpster.com/resources/how-to-declutter-your-home.php

Bulkeley, K. (2019). *Keeping a Dream Journal*. Psychology Today. https://www.psychologytoday.com/ca/blog/dreaming-in-the-digital-age/201705/keeping-dream-journal

Bullet Journal. (2020). *Learn*. Bullet Journal. https://bulletjournal.com/pages/learn

Burns, M. (2014, February 17). *5 Steps to Declutter Your Schedule and Live Your Desired Life*. Becoming Minimalist. https://www.becomingminimalist.com/declutter-your-schedule/

Carrico, M. (2007, August 28). *A Beginner's Guide to Meditation*. Yoga Journal; Yoga Journal. https://www.yogajournal.com/meditation/let-s-meditate/

Carstens-Peters, G. (2017a, January 15). *person writing bucket list on book*. Unsplash.com; Unsplash. https://unsplash.com/photos/RLw-UC03Gwc

Carstens-Peters, G. (2017b, February 5). *person using MacBook Pro*. Unsplash.com; Unsplash. https://unsplash.com/photos/npxXWgQ33ZQ

CDC. (2020, February 11). *What Workers and Employers Can Do to Manage Workplace Fatigue during COVID-19*. Centers for Disease Control and Prevention. https://www.cdc.gov/coronavirus/2019-ncov/hcp/managing-workplace-fatigue.html

Cherry, K. (2021a). *How Does Self-Determination Theory Explain Motivation?* Verywell Mind. https://www.verywellmind.com/what-is-self-determination-theory-2795387#:~:text=In%20psychology%2C%20self%2Ddetermination%20is,over%20their%20choices%20and%20lives.

Cherry, K. (2021b). *How Does Self-Determination Theory Explain Motivation?* Verywell Mind. https://www.verywellmind.com/what-is-self-determination-theory-2795387#:~:text=In%20psychology%2C%20self%2Ddetermination%20is,over%20their%20choices%20and%20lives.

Clave-Brule, M., Mazloum, A., Park, R. J., Harbottle, E. J., & Birmingham, C. L. (2009). Managing anxiety in eating disorders with knitting. *Eating and Weight Disorders - Studies on Anorexia, Bulimia and Obesity, 14*(1), e1–e5. https://doi.org/10.1007/bf03354620

Clear, J. (2020, November 26). *The Clear Habit Journal.* James Clear. https://jamesclear.com/habit-journal

Cleveland Clinic. (2021). *Chronic Illness: Sources of Stress, How to Cope.* Cleveland Clinic. https://my.clevelandclinic.org/health/articles/4062-chronic-illness

Connley, C. (2018, September 13). *Here's what making your bed (or not) reveals about your personality.* CNBC; CNBC. https://www.cnbc.com/2018/09/12/heres-what-making-your-bed-or-not-reveals-about-your-personality.html#:~:text=%E2%80%9CIf%20you%20make%20your%20bed,turned%20into%20many%20tasks%20completed.%E2%80%9D

Conscious Design. (2020, July 3). *woman in brown knit sweater holding brown ceramic cup.* Unsplash.com; Unsplash. https://unsplash.com/photos/VsI_74zRzAo

Cook, J. (2007, August 28). *Find Your Match Among the Many Types of Yoga.* Yoga Journal; Yoga Journal. https://www.yogajournal.com/practice/not-all-yoga-is-created-equal/

Cronkleton, E. (2019, April 9). *10 Breathing Techniques for Stress Relief and More.* Healthline; Healthline Media. https://www.healthline.com/health/breathing-exercise#sitali-breath

Daily Stoic. (2018, July). *What Is Stoicism? A Definition & 9 Stoic Exercises To Get You Started.* Daily Stoic. https://dailystoic.com/what-is-stoicism-a-definition-3-stoic-exercises-to-get-you-started/

Danielle, M. (2017, August 28). *The History of Minimalism And What Minimalism Means as a Lifestyle.* Mia Danielle. https://miadanielle.com/what-is-minimalism/

Davis, N. (2019, September 24). *30 Moves to Make the Most of Your At-Home Workout.* Healthline; Healthline Media. https://www.healthline.com/health/fitness-exercise/at-home-workouts#beginner-routine

Davis, T. (2020). *4 New Ways to Find Meaning and Purpose.* Psychology Today. https://www.psychologytoday.com/us/blog/click-here-happiness/202008/4-new-ways-find-meaning-and-purpose

Debret, C. (2019, February). *A History of The Great American Food Pyramid and How to Make Better Choices Today!* One Green Planet; One Green Planet. https://www.onegreenplanet.org/natural-health/history-of-the-food-pyramid-plant-based/

Devaney, E. (2021, June 8). *How to Work From Home: 24 Tips From People Who Do It Successfully.* Hubspot.com. https://blog.hubspot.com/marketing/productivity-tips-working-from-home

Donnelly, M. (2018, July 30). *Just As You Are, You Are Enough | Word & Sole.* Word & Sole. https://wordandsole.com/just-as-you-are-you-are-enough/

Duffy, J. (2015, March 11). *20 Tips for Working From Home.* PCMAG; PCMag. https://www.pcmag.com/news/get-organized-20-tips-for-working-from-home

Dutta, S. (2010, November). *Managing Yourself: What's Your Personal Social Media Strategy?* Harvard Business Review. https://hbr.org/2010/11/managing-yourself-whats-your-personal-social-media-strategy

Earley, B. (2020, February 4). *The 5 Love Languages and Their Meanings.* Oprah.com; Oprah.com. https://www.oprah.com/relationships/the-5-love-languages-and-their-meanings

Effectiviology. (2011). *FOMO: How to Overcome the Fear of Missing Out – Effectiviology.*

Effectiviology.com. https://effectiviology.com/fomo-the-fear-of-missing-out/

Effectiviology. (2016). *The Dangers of Social Media and How to Avoid Them – Effectiviology.* Effectiviology.com. https://effectiviology.com/dangers-of-social-media/

Eurich, T. (2018a, January 4). *What Self-Awareness Really Is (and How to Cultivate It).* Harvard Business Review. https://hbr.org/2018/01/what-self-awareness-really-is-and-how-to-cultivate-it

Eurich, T. (2018b, January 4). *What Self-Awareness Really Is (and How to Cultivate It).* Harvard Business Review. https://hbr.org/2018/01/what-self-awareness-really-is-and-how-to-cultivate-it

Fader, S. (2020a, December 11). *10 Daily Self-Care Activities | Betterhelp.* Betterhelp.com; BetterHelp. https://www.betterhelp.com/advice/mindfulness/10-daily-self-care-activities/

Fader, S. (2020b, December 11). *10 Daily Self-Care Activities | Betterhelp.* Betterhelp.com; BetterHelp. https://www.betterhelp.com/advice/mindfulness/10-daily-self-care-activities/

Fader, S. (2020c, December 11). *A Simple Introduction To Mindfulness | Betterhelp.* Betterhelp.com; BetterHelp. https://www.betterhelp.com/advice/mindfulness/a-simple-introduction-to-mindfulness/

Fader, S. (2020d, December 11). *A Simple Introduction To Mindfulness | Betterhelp.* Betterhelp.com; BetterHelp. https://www.betterhelp.com/advice/mindfulness/a-simple-introduction-to-mindfulness/

Fader, S. (2020e, December 11). *An Easy To Follow Self-Care Guide | Betterhelp.* Betterhelp.com; BetterHelp. https://www.betterhelp.com/advice/mindfulness/an-easy-to-follow-self-care-guide/

Fader, S. (2020f, December 11). *Basic Self-Care Tips For Beginners | Betterhelp.* Betterhelp.com; BetterHelp. https://www.betterhelp.com/advice/mindfulness/basic-self-care-tips-for-beginners/

Fader, S. (2020g, December 11). *Basic Self-Care Tips For Beginners | Betterhelp.* Betterhelp.com; BetterHelp. https://www.betterhelp.com/advice/mindfulness/basic-self-care-tips-for-beginners/

Fields, J. (2019, December 27). *Play the 30-Day Minimalism Game.* The Minimalists; The Minimalists. https://www.theminimalists.com/game/

Foster, B. L. (2015, June 11). *How to Master Working From Home—While Under Quarantine With Kids.* Parents; Parents. https://www.parents.com/parenting/work/life-balance/how-to-master-being-a-work-at-home-mom/

Freemind, S. (2018, August 15). *man standing in front of the window.* Unsplash.com; Unsplash. https://unsplash.com/photos/Pv5WeEyxMWU

Gaiam. (2020). *Meditation 101: Techniques, Benefits, and a Beginner's How-to.* Gaiam. https://www.gaiam.com/blogs/discover/meditation-101-techniques-benefits-and-a-beginner-s-how-to

Garis, M. G. (2019, October 29). *There are 4 types of intimacy, and only 1 includes touching.* Well+Good. https://www.wellandgood.com/types-of-intimacy/

Garrity, A. (2019, January 11). *What Is the KonMari Method? Here's How to Declutter the Marie Kondo Way.* Good Housekeeping; Good Housekeeping. https://www.goodhousekeeping.com/home/organizing/a25846191/what-is-the-konmari-method/

Gaskill, L. (2016, January 8). How To Keep Surfaces Clutter-Free. *Forbes.* https://www.forbes.com/sites/houzz/2016/01/08/how-to-keep-surfaces-clutter-free/?sh=370f19753a62

Gerhardt, N. (2021, March 20). *10 Things to Know About Swedish Death Cleaning.* Family Handyman; Family Handyman. https://www.familyhandyman.com/list/10-things-to-know-about-swedish-death-cleaning/

GoodTherapy. (2013). *Intimacy.* GoodTherapy Blog. https://www.goodtherapy.org/blog/psychpedia/intimacy

Gorman, S., & Gorman, J. M. (2020). *Is Information Overload Hurting Mental Health?* Psychology Today. https://www.psychologytoday.com/us/blog/denying-the-grave/202006/is-information-overload-hurting-mental-health#:~:text=Information%20overload%20can%20lead%20to,hasty%20(often%20bad)%20decisions.

Gottardi, C. (2016, June 29). *A woman walking through a forest in the afternoon.* Unsplash.com; Unsplash. https://unsplash.com/photos/p5JVzahHku0

Harbinger, A. J. (2018, October 26). *Signs of a Toxic Person | How to Cut Toxic People from Your Life.* The Art of Charm. https://theartofcharm.com/art-of-personal-development/empowerment/cut-toxic-people-life/

Harvard Health Publishing. (2005, September 30). *10 steps for coping with a chronic condition - Harvard Health.* Harvard Health; Harvard Health. https://www.health.harvard.edu/staying-healthy/10-steps-for-coping-with-a-chronic-condition

Harvard Health Publishing. (2015, January 26). *Relaxation techniques: Breath control helps quell errant stress response - Harvard Health.* Harvard Health; Harvard Health. https://www.health.harvard.edu/mind-and-mood/relaxation-techniques-breath-control-helps-quell-errant-stress-response

Hassan, P. (2017, June 11). *man looking at the skies.* Unsplash.com; Unsplash. https://unsplash.com/photos/0E1PYojm4CY

Headspace. (2021a). *Meditation for Beginners.* Headspace. https://www.headspace.com/meditation/meditation-for-beginners

Headspace. (2021b). *What are all the types of meditation & which one is best?* Headspace. https://www.headspace.com/meditation/techniques

Henderson, A. (2019, January 22). *9 easy ways to make your house feel homey | Style at Home.* Style at Home. https://www.styleathome.com/how-to/tips-and-tricks/article/9-easy-ways-to-make-your-house-feel-homey

Henry, J. (2019, June 25). *What Does "You Are Enough" Mean? - The Startup - Medium.* Medium; The Startup. https://medium.com/swlh/what-does-you-are-enough-mean-e166d47b0673

Hurst, K. (2016, July 13). *Removing Toxic People From Your Life In 9 Steps.* The Law of Attraction. https://www.thelawofattraction.com/removing-toxic-people-life/

Inlanta Mortgage. (2020, December). *14 Ways to Make Your Home Cozy and Inviting - Inlanta Mortgage.* Inlanta Mortgage. https://www.inlanta.com/14-ways-cozy-home/

Jaret, P. (2010, May 21). *9 Ways to Get Your Energy Back.* WebMD; WebMD. https://www.webmd.com/balance/features/get-energy-back

Jimenez, C. (2019, November 7). *people using phone while standing.* Unsplash.com; Unsplash. https://unsplash.com/photos/qZenO_gQ7QA

Johnson, M. (2019, April 16). *How to Understand and Build Intimacy in Every Relationship.* Healthline; Healthline Media. https://www.healthline.com/health/intimacy#different-types

Journey. (2021). *Journey.Cloud - Free Online Journal & Diary.* Journey.Cloud. https://journey.cloud/journaling-benefits/

Juddblog. (2018, August 13). *10 Ways to Make Your House More Welcoming to You...* Juddbuilders.com; Judd Builders. https://www.juddbuilders.com/juddbuildersblog/2018/08/13/10-ways-to-make-your-house-more-welcoming-to-your-guests/

Kettering University Online. (2019, April 15). *Why Hobbies Are Important?* Kettering.edu. https://online.kettering.edu/news/2019/04/15/why-hobbies-are-important

Klahre, A.-M. (2019, September 16). *9 Easy Ways to Cozy Up Your Home.* Real Simple; Real Simple. https://www.realsimple.com/home-organizing/easy-ways-cozy-home

Kleidon, K. (2018, July 17). *11 Habits of Minimalist Living You Can Adopt Today.* Project Hot Mess. https://projecthotmess.com/habits-of-minimalist-living/

Klein, A. (2018, July 23). *round grey moon chair with brown pillow on top.* Unsplash.com; Unsplash. https://unsplash.com/photos/JaXs8Tk5Iww

Kondo, M. (2019a, April). *How to Greet Your Home – KonMari | The Official Website of Marie Kondo.* KonMari | The Official Website of Marie Kondo. https://konmari.com/how-to-greet-your-home/

Kondo, M. (2019b, November 12). *6 Ways to Purify Your Space – KonMari | The Official Website of Marie Kondo.* KonMari | The Official Website of Marie Kondo. https://konmari.com/home-purification/

Kondo, M. (2020a, March 12). *Marie's Self-Care Practices – KonMari | The Official Website of Marie Kondo.* KonMari | The Official Website of Marie Kondo. https://konmari.com/marie-kondo-meditation/

Kondo, M. (2020b, July 23). *Guided Meditation With Marie – KonMari | The Official Website of Marie Kondo.* KonMari | The Official Website of Marie Kondo. https://konmari.com/guided-meditation-marie-kondo/

Krans, B. (2015, March 23). *Foods That Beat Fatigue.* Healthline; Healthline Media. https://www.healthline.com/health/food-nutrition/foods-that-beat-fatigue#fruits-and-vegetables

Krstic, Z. (2021, January 15). *The Best Diets of 2021, According to Our Registered Dietitian.* Good Housekeeping; Good Housekeeping. https://www.goodhousekeeping.com/health/diet-nutrition/a35217200/best-diets-2021/

Kurtz, J. L. (2015). *Six Reasons to Get a Hobby.* Psychology Today. https://www.psychologytoday.com/ca/blog/happy-trails/201509/six-reasons-get-hobby

Lane, E. (2018). *33 of the Best Beginner Exercises to Sweat Through During Home Workouts.* Men's Health; Men's Health. https://www.menshealth.com/uk/building-muscle/a754099/the-15-best-beginners-exercises-to-do-at-home/

Langevin, M. (2021, February 4). *white ceramic mug on white table.* Unsplash.com; Unsplash. https://unsplash.com/photos/bg4Vz54j9x8

Lawler, M. (2020, April 5). *How to Start a Self-Care Routine You'll Follow | Everyday Health.* EverydayHealth.com. https://www.everydayhealth.com/self-care/start-a-self-care-routine/

Le Minh Phuong. (2017, December 12). *a woman meditating on wooden dock during daytime.* Unsplash.com; Unsplash. https://unsplash.com/photos/niH7Z81S44g

Lee, D. J. (2014, October 27). 6 Tips For Better Work-Life Balance. *Forbes.* https://www.forbes.com/sites/deborahlee/2014/10/20/6-tips-for-better-work-life-balance/?sh=5dde0be929ff

Lifford, J. (2017, August 29). *The 30 Day Home Decluttering Detox Plan.* Oprah.com; Oprah.com. https://www.oprah.com/home/the-30-day-home-decluttering-detox-plan_1

Lindberg, S. (2019, August 7). *13 Brain Exercises to Help Keep You Mentally Sharp.* Healthline; Healthline Media. https://www.healthline.com/health/mental-health/brain-exercises#play-cards

Lucy. (2019, November 14). *Reasons Why Home Decoration is Important» Residence Style.* Residence Style. https://www.residencestyle.com/reasons-why-home-decoration-is-important/

MacMillan, A. (2017, October 17). *"Death Cleaning" Is the Newest Way to Declutter. Here's What to Know.* Time; Time. https://time.com/4985533/death-cleaning-declutter/

Madell, R. (2012, October 19). *Battling the Stress of Living with Chronic Illness.* Healthline; Healthline Media. https://www.healthline.com/health/depression/chronic-illness

Maertz, Dr. K. (2019). *Strategies To Build Healthy Self-Esteem.* https://www.mcgill.ca/counselling/files/counselling/self-esteem_helpful_hints_0.pdf

Making Lemonade. (2016, January 11). *The Ultimate FREE Printable Decluttering Checklist for KonMari Success! - Making Lemonade.* Making Lemonade. https://makinglemonadeblog.com/free-printable-decluttering-konmari-method-checklist/

Making Lemonade. (2019, November 19). *It's Here! Get Your FREE 2020 Printable Planner! - Making Lemonade.* Making Lemonade: Your Life, Organized. https://makinglemonadeblog.com/free-2020-printable-planner-pretty-modern-farmhouse/

Marcel, G. (2016, June 19). *four people sitting on wooden stair.* Unsplash.com; Unsplash. https://unsplash.com/photos/AWidiBoRO08

Marr, B. (2015, November 25). Why Too Much Data Is Stressing Us Out. *Forbes.* https://www.forbes.com/sites/bernardmarr/2015/11/25/why-too-much-data-is-stressing-us-out/?sh=20536ffbf763

Mayo Clinic Staff. (2020a). *A beginner's guide to meditation.* Mayo Clinic; https://www.mayoclinic.org/tests-procedures/meditation/in-depth/meditation/art-20045858

Mayo Clinic Staff. (2020b). *Tips to regain your work-life balance.* Mayo Clinic; https://www.mayoclinic.org/healthy-lifestyle/adult-health/in-depth/work-life-balance/art-20048134

Mayo Clinic Staff. (2021a). *Herbal supplements: What to know before you buy.* Mayo Clinic; https://www.mayoclinic.org/healthy-lifestyle/nutrition-and-healthy-eating/in-depth/herbal-supplements/art-20046714

Mayo Clinic Staff. (2021b). *The truth behind the most popular diet trends of the moment.* Mayo Clinic; https://www.mayoclinic.org/healthy-lifestyle/weight-loss/in-depth/the-truth-behind-the-most-popular-diet-trends-of-the-moment/art-20390062

Mayo Clinic Staff. (2021c). *The truth behind the most popular diet trends of the moment.* Mayo Clinic; https://www.mayoclinic.org/healthy-lifestyle/weight-loss/in-depth/the-truth-behind-the-most-popular-diet-trends-of-the-moment/art-20390062

McAlary, B. (2014, December 9). *Don't know what stuff to keep? Have a packing party! – Slow Your Home.* Slowyourhome.com. https://slowyourhome.com/packing-party/#:~:text=Essentially%2C%20the%20idea%20is%20to,or%20toss%20the%20unused%20items.

McDonough, L. S., & Picard, C. (2016, March 22). *The Ultimate Cleaning Schedule for Your Day, Week, Month, and Year.* Good Housekeeping; Good Housekeeping. https://www.goodhousekeeping.com/home/cleaning/a37462/how-often-you-should-clean-everything/

Mead, E. (2019, September 26). *What is Positive Self-Talk? (Incl. Examples).* PositivePsychology.com. https://positivepsychology.com/positive-self-talk/

Merriam-Webster. (2021). Intimacy. In *Merriam-webster.com.* https://www.merriam-webster.com/dictionary/intimate

Miah, E. (2017, January 31). *6 Reasons you should re-decorate your house.* YourStory.com; Yourstory. https://yourstory.com/mystory/badcacdc94-6-reasons-you-should-re-decorate-your-house/amp

Migala, J. (2020, April 30). *5 Ways a Skin-Care Routine Benefits Mental Health | Everyday Health.* EverydayHealth.com. https://www.everydayhealth.com/skin-beauty/5-reasons-maintaining-a-skin-care-routine-is-good-for-your-mental-health/

Mind Tool Content Team. (2017). *Building Self-Confidence: Preparing Yourself for Success.* Mindtools.com. https://www.mindtools.com/selfconf.html

Minimalism. (2019, January 9). *Self-care tips: 11 self-care activities to build into your routine.* Minimalism. https://minimalism.co/articles/self-care-routine

Minimalism Made Simple. (2020, June 21). *15 Reasons to Believe You Are Enough.* Minimalism Made Simple. https://www.minimalismmadesimple.com/home/you-are-enough/

Montgomery, C. (2020, April 29). *macbook pro displaying group of people.* Unsplash.com; Unsplash. https://unsplash.com/photos/smgTvepind4

Moran, G. (2020, March 2). *How to use a bullet journal to kick-start your mindfulness practice.* Fast Company; Fast Company. https://www.fastcompany.com/90469534/how-to-use-a-bullet-journal-to-kickstart-your-mindfulness-practice

Neff, K. (2020a, July 9). *Definition and Three Elements of Self Compassion.* Self-Compassion. https://self-compassion.org/the-three-elements-of-self-compassion-2/

Neff, K. (2020b, July 9). *Definition and Three Elements of Self Compassion.* Self-Compassion. https://self-compassion.org/the-three-elements-of-self-compassion-2/

NeONBRAND. (2018, March 10). *two person holding black and red ceramic mugs.* Unsplash.com; Unsplash. https://unsplash.com/photos/u4M4JezA7uM

Nicodemus, R. (2014, December 4). *Packing Party: Unpack a Simpler Life.* The Minimalists; The Minimalists. https://www.theminimalists.com/packing/

Nothingam, S. (2013, September 25). *10 Feng Shui Tips For A Happy And Harmonious Home.* Decoist; Decoist. https://www.decoist.com/2013-09-25/feng-shui-tips/?edg-c=1

O'Connell, K. (2012, September 10). *Causes of Fatigue and How to Manage It.* Healthline; Healthline Media. https://www.healthline.com/health/fatigue

Olsson, E. (2019, January 15). *vegetable salad.* Unsplash.com; Unsplash. https://unsplash.com/photos/KPDbRyFOTnE

Online Etymology Dictionary. (2021). Meditation. In *Online Etymology Dictionary.* https://www.etymonline.com/word/meditation

Organize with Ease. (2019, April 18). *Decluttering Challenge: How I Failed the 30-Day Minimalism Game.* Organize with Ease. https://slowmotionmama.com/30-day-minimalism-game/

Organized Sparkle. (2020, May 2). *Two Decluttering Methods Explored KonMari vs 4 Boxes | Organized Sparkle.* Organized Sparkle. https://organizedsparkle.com/decluttering-methods/

Oron, S. (2018, April 17). *The Importance of Finding Your Own Enough in This Lifetime.* Medium; The Startup. https://medium.com/swlh/what-happens-when-you-find-your-enough-in-this-lifetime-65fdc4844aa6

Osmond, A. (2021, March 24). *Write a bucket list to improve physical and mental health.* Daily Herald. https://www.heraldextra.com/lifestyles/health-and-fitness/write-a-bucket-list-to-improve-physical-and-mental-health/article_29cf4ce6-1fbb-5cf7-8013-1494529557d5.html

Parker-Pope, T. (2021). How to Find a Hobby. *The New York Times*. https://www.nytimes.com/guides/smarterliving/how-to-find-a-hobby

Pasternack, A. (2019, June 16). *How to use social media, according to a mental health expert.* Fast Company; Fast Company. https://www.fastcompany.com/90356260/social-media-can-hurt-you-these-6-tips-from-a-psychologist-could-help

Patterson, R. (2019, September 10). *The 11 Best Habit Tracking Apps in 2021.* College Info Geek. https://collegeinfogeek.com/habit-tracker/

Perera, A. (2020, September 4). *Self-Actualization | Simply Psychology.* Simplypsychology.org. https://www.simplypsychology.org/self-actualization.html#:~:text=Self%2Dactualization%20is%20the%20complete,every%20human%20being%20reaches%20it.

Perkins, M. S. (2017, September 11). *I took the 30-day minimalism challenge, got rid of 338 possessions, and still failed — here's what I learned.* Business Insider; Business Insider. https://www.businessinsider.com/30-day-minimalism-challenge-how-to-downsize-your-life-2017-8

Phillips, L. (2018, November 28). *The Best Daily, Weekly, and Monthly Planners to Make 2021 Your Most Organized Year Yet.* Real Simple; Real Simple. https://www.realsimple.com/work-life/life-strategies/planner-agenda-daily-weekly-monthly

Pinola, M. (2019, January 3). *The 8 best journal apps of 2021.* Zapier.com; Zapier. https://zapier.com/blog/best-journaling-apps/

Raypole, C. (2020a, May 28). *5 Visualization Techniques to Add to Your Meditation Practice.* Healthline; Healthline Media. https://www.healthline.com/health/visualization-meditation

Raypole, C. (2020b, August 17). *6 Ways Friendship Is Good for Your Health.* Healthline; Healthline Media. https://www.healthline.com/health/benefits-of-friendship

Rodriguez, R. (2018). *The Four Box Method – Decluttering – ADHD Center for Success.* Adhdcenterforsuccess.com. https://adhdcenterforsuccess.com/site/the-four-box-method-decluttering/

Rooney, J. (2020, October 23). *The Importance of Self-Care - Tri-State Memorial Hospital.* Tri-State Memorial Hospital. https://tristatehospital.org/the-importance-of-self-care/

Rutledge, P. B. (2016). *The Pressures of Social Media: Should I Disconnect?* Psychology Today. https://www.psychologytoday.com/ca/blog/positively-media/201607/the-pressures-social-media-should-i-disconnect

Sangerma, E. (2020, August 28). *Why Keep a Dream Journal - Publishous - Medium.* Medium; Publishous. https://medium.com/publishous/why-keep-a-dream-journal-5c66913fcd3c

Sass, C. (2021, January 4). *The Best (and Worst) Diets for 2021, According to Experts.* Health.com; Health.com. https://www.health.com/weight-loss/best-diets-2021

Scott, E. (2021). *How to Enjoy Your Life by Making a Bucket List.* Verywell Mind. https://www.verywellmind.com/benefits-of-a-bucket-list-3144998#:~:text=Creating%20a%20bucket%20list%20can%20help%20you%20tap%20into%20the,dreams%20and%20plans%20into%20action.

Silverthorne, N. (2020, April 3). *11 tips for working from home with kids around that ACTUALLY work.* Today's Parent. https://www.todaysparent.com/family/family-life/working-from-home-with-kids-coronavirus/

Simple Living. (2020, September 15). *Types of Minimalists | Frugal, Sustainable, Nomad | Which one are you?* Minimalism. https://minimalism.co/articles/types-of-minimalists

Sissons, C. (2020, July 27). *Useful breathing techniques to consider trying.* Medicalnewstoday.com; Medical News Today. https://www.medicalnewstoday.com/articles/breathing-techniques#pursed-lip

Sixteen Miles Out. (2020, April 8). *white notebook on white textile.* Unsplash.com; Unsplash. https://unsplash.com/photos/3ZvHsFiZyME

Smart Garden Guide. (2019a, July 2). *37 Small Indoor Plants To Bring Beauty Into Your Home - Smart Garden Guide.* Smart Garden Guide. https://smartgardenguide.com/small-indoor-plants/#:~:text=37%20Small%20Indoor%20Plants%20To%20Bring%20Beauty%20Into,Chinese%20Money%20Plant%20%28Pilea%20Peperomiodes%29%20More%20items...%20

Smart Garden Guide. (2019b, July 2). *37 Small Indoor Plants To Bring Beauty Into Your Home - Smart Garden Guide.* Smart Garden Guide. https://smartgardenguide.com/small-indoor-plants/#:~:text=37%20Small%20Indoor%20Plants%20To%20Bring%20Beauty%20Into,Chinese%20Money%20Plant%20%28Pilea%20Peperomiodes%29%20More%20items...%20

Smith, I. (2018, December 14). *three pens on white paper.* Unsplash.com; Unsplash. https://unsplash.com/photos/8XlMU62ii8I

Socialist Health Association. (2019a, February 14). *The best and worst common indoor plants for allergy sufferers.* Socialist Health Association. https://www.sochealth.co.uk/sp/health/the-best-and-worst-common-indoor-plants-for-allergy-sufferers/

Socialist Health Association. (2019b, February 14). *The best and worst common indoor plants for allergy sufferers.* Socialist Health Association. https://www.sochealth.co.uk/sp/health/the-best-and-worst-common-indoor-plants-for-allergy-sufferers/

Spritzler, F. (2019, April 29). *29 Healthy Snacks That Can Help You Lose Weight.* Healthline; Healthline Media. https://www.healthline.com/nutrition/29-healthy-snacks-for-weight-loss

Surban, G. (2018, February 19). *22 Benefits of Having a Hobby or Enjoying a Leisure Activity.* Develop Good Habits. https://www.developgoodhabits.com/benefits-hobby/

The Positivity Project. (2021, May 10). *Positive Psychology's 24 Character Strengths.* The Positivity Project. https://posproject.org/character-strengths/

Thorpe, M. (2020, October 26). *12 Science-Based Benefits of Meditation.* Healthline; Healthline Media. https://www.healthline.com/nutrition/12-benefits-of-meditation#8.-May-help-fight-addictions

Thought Catalog. (2019, April 12). *blooming yellow gerbera daisy flower in white and black mug.* Unsplash.com; Unsplash. https://unsplash.com/photos/Ecnx13MEPK0

TNN. (2015, December 26). *Advantages of deep breathing exercises.* The Times of India; Times Of India. https://timesofindia.indiatimes.com/life-style/health-fitness/fitness/advantages-of-deep-breathing-exercises/articleshow/19213960.cms

Tu, T. (2017, July 27). *gray dress shirt hang on brown wooden rack in front of window with white curtain.* Unsplash.com; Unsplash. https://unsplash.com/photos/QZGQO3NvsLo

Turner, C. (2020, April). *Tall Indoor Plants | 7 Best Large Houseplants to Grow in Your Home - My Tasteful Space.* My Tasteful Space. https://blog.mytastefulspace.com/2020/04/01/tall-indoor-plants/

Urban Dictionary. (2019). Snaccident. In *Urban Dictionary.* https://www.urbandictionary.com/define.php?term=Snaccident

US News. (2021). *Best Diets Overall.* Usnews.com. https://health.usnews.com/best-diet/best-diets-overall

Van, G. (2018, May 28). *11 Vitamins and Supplements That Boost Energy.* Healthline; Healthline Media.

https://www.healthline.com/nutrition/best-supplements-for-energy

Vanilla Papers. (2020, August 25). *13 Powerful Journaling Techniques (And How To Start)*. Vanilla Papers. https://vanillapapers.net/2020/08/25/journaling-techniques/

Vivien. (2019, February 20). *7 Secrets To Creating a Cozy Home | Posh Pennies*. Posh Pennies. https://poshpennies.com/how-to-make-a-cozy-home/

Wanjek, C. (2014, June 2). *Learning a New Language at Any Age Helps the Brain*. Livescience.com; Live Science. https://www.livescience.com/46048-learning-new-language-brain.html

Weiner, Z. (2017, March 22). *7 Tips for Eliminating Toxic People From Your Life*. Mentalfloss.com. https://www.mentalfloss.com/article/93521/7-tips-eliminating-toxic-people-your-life

Westbury. (2019, August 15). *The health benefits of natural light and space in the home - Westbury Garden Rooms*. Westbury Garden Rooms. https://www.westburygardenrooms.com/blog/health-benefits-natural-light-and-space/

White, A. (2021, May 17). *1000+ Bucket List Ideas: The Best Things to Do Before You Die*. Bucket List Journey | Travel + Lifestyle Blog. https://bucketlistjourney.net/my-bucket-list/

Wilkins, M. C. (2015, August 3). *5 Types of Minimalism*. No Sidebar. https://nosidebar.com/types-of-minimalist/

Wong, C. (2021). *Learn How to Make a Mindfulness Meditation Practice Part of Your Day*. Verywell Mind. https://www.verywellmind.com/mindfulness-meditation-88369

Yankovich, G. (2018, April). *A Beginner's Guide To Swedish Death Cleaning*. BuzzFeed. https://www.buzzfeed.com/gyanyankovich/what-is-swedish-death-cleaning

Yarrow, K. (2014, November 20). *12 Ways to Stop Wasting Money and Take Control of Your Stuff*. Money; Money. https://money.com/overspending-overconsumption-stuff/

Your Visual Journal. (2019, March 12). *How to Journal | The Ultimate Guide*. Your Visual Journal. https://yourvisualjournal.com/how-to-journal-the-ultimate-guide/

Yuko, E. (2020, April 24). *The Pros and Cons of a Made Bed*. Architectural Digest; Architectural Digest. https://www.architecturaldigest.com/story/pros-and-cons-of-a-made-bed

Zaki, Y. (2017, September 9). *The dangers of social media that no one likes to admit*. Gulfnews.com; Gulf News. https://gulfnews.com/opinion/op-eds/the-dangers-of-social-media-that-no-one-likes-to-admit-1.2087285

Zamora, D. (2004, September 16). *Foods to Fight Fatigue*. WebMD; WebMD. https://www.webmd.com/food-recipes/features/foods-fight-fatigue

Made in United States
North Haven, CT
23 November 2022

27152302R00053